THE MOST WIDELY ACCLAIMED AND INFORMATIVE BOOK ON THE AIDS EPIDEMIC

"Engagingly written"
 —The Advocate

"Easy to read . . . of great value to everyone involved in protecting the health of the community."
 —**Florence Seibert, Ph.D., Professor Emeritus, University of Pennsylvania**

"Cantwell has done his homework."
 —**The Los Angeles Times Book Review**

"Cantwell's book is like Norman Cousins' *Anatomy of an Illness* in that it explores the effects of psychology on illnesses and questions many assumptions of the medical profession about the nature and causes of illness."
 —**The Small Press Book Review**

"A daring, exciting, and provocative book. I urge everyone interested in AIDS to read this remarkable book . . . it will stimulate your thinking."
 —**Armand Auger, M.D., Los Angeles**

"As one of America's preeminent researchers into the microbiology of cancer, Doctor Cantwell has produced a highly readable and scientifically sound volume on one of the most terrifying syndromes of our time. This definitive book is a must-read for anyone interested in finding out the truth about AIDS, instead of relying on front-page hysterics for their information. The highest of marks for Cantwell and this long-overdue, fascinating book!"
 —**Ed Addeo, Co-author of "The Conquest of Cancer"**

ARIES RISING PRESS
P.O. BOX 29532
LOS ANGELES CA 90029
58
69

D1206236

AIDS:
THE MYSTERY
AND THE SOLUTION

AIDS:
THE MYSTERY
AND
THE SOLUTION

Alan Cantwell, Jr., M.D.

SECOND EDITION, REVISED

ARIES RISING PRESS

Los Angeles

The material contained in this book is not meant to be a manual for self-diagnosis, or self treatment, nor should it be a substitute for the advice of a medical doctor.

Library of Congress Cataloging-in-Publication Data

Cantwell, Alan, 1934-
    AIDS: The Mystery and the Solution.

    Includes bibliographies and indexes
    1. Acquired immune deficiency syndrome. 1. Title
[DNLM: 1. Acquired immune deficiency syndrome.
RC607.A26C36   1986   616.9'7'92   86-1210

ISBN 0-917211-08-1 (hardcover)

ISBN 0-917211-16-2 (paperback)

To Virginia Livingston, M.D.

who showed me the way

and

To Frank A. Sinatra

who kept me on the path

"*The question of epidemics cannot be answered from a biological standpoint alone. It involves great sweeping psychological attitudes on the part of many, and meets the needs and desires of those involved — needs which arise in the framework of religious, psychological, and cultural realities that cannot be isolated from biological traits.*"

"*On one level the deaths are a protest against the time in which they occur. Those involved have private reasons, however. The reasons, of course, vary from one individual to another, yet all involved 'want their death to serve a purpose' beyond private concerns. Partially, then, such deaths are meant to make the survivors question the conditions — for unconsciously the species well knows there are reasons for such mass deaths that go beyond accepted beliefs.*"

—Jane Roberts, The Individual and the Nature of Mass Events. A Seth Book. (1981).

ACKNOWLEDGEMENT

During the past twenty years as a medical doctor and scientific researcher, there have been many people who have greatly stimulated my thoughts about human disease. However, none of my research into the microbiology of cancer and collagen disease could have originated without the help of Eugenia Craggs, a bacteriologist, who first taught me how to patiently and painstakingly hunt for microbes in diseased tissue. She also taught me to respect the unusual microbes she grew from diseased tissue in her tuberculosis (TB) laboratory, and to consider these bacteria as possible agents of human disease, even though these microbes were isolated from diseases "of unknown etiology."

I am especially grateful to my friends, Virginia Livingston Wheeler, M.D., Eleanor Alexander-Jackson, Irene Corey Diller, and Florence Seibert, for sharing their knowledge of the "cancer microbe" with me. Their landmark studies of the microbiology of cancer have influenced my own research studies immeasurably. Other microbiologists who have greatly stimulated my thinking about "cell wall deficient bacteria" include Lida Mattman, Gerald Domingue, Dan Kelso, and Joyce Jones. Pathologists who have been especially helpful include Karen Cove, M.D., and Jerry Lawson, M.D.

My research studies over the past three decades could not have been successful without the support of my "boss," Lyon Rowe, M.D., and Sheldon Wolf, M.D., who often fought in my behalf, to secure continuing grant money to support my research projects.

Researchers must "publish or perish." Editors of medical journals who have been most kind in helping me attain scientific "credibility" include the following editors: Gardner Moment (*GROWTH*), Lawrence Charles Parish (*International Journal of Dermatology*), Eugene Traub and John McCarthy (*CUTIS*), and Frederick Malkinson (*Archives of Dermatology*).

Judy Dowd, Linda Yamamoto, Winnie Yu, and Jeff Elser helped greatly in securing the reference material in this book. During the writing of this book, Armand Auger, M.D., provided much-needed encouragement, and Jim Highland made many helpful suggestions in the editing of the manuscript.

Larry Gosenfeld, D.O., gave me the idea of writing this book on a computer word-processor. The manuscript was written on an "Apple 2E," and printed on a "Gemini 10" printer, both of which served me faithfully and admirably, and deserve to be acknowledged as a writer's best friends.

Finally, I am most greatly indebted to my patients for allowing me to study them. The courage often shown by patients, especially those seriously ill with cancer, and AIDS, has contributed immeasurably to bolstering my own courage, and my determination to share what I have learned about these diseases with others.

TABLE OF CONTENTS

INTRODUCTION

AIDS is an acronym which stands for the Acquired Immune Deficiency Syndrome. By definition, all persons with AIDS have weakened or damaged "immune systems." At present, medical scientists do not know how or why these immune system abnormalities are "acquired" in AIDS. But one thing is certain. Cancer and serious "opportunistic" infections often develop as a result of the immunodeficiency in AIDS.

The results of epidemiologic studies suggest that AIDS is both infectious and contagious, and may be transmitted through sexual intercourse. In addition, the suspected infectious agent may be spread through blood transfusions or blood products. This possible blood-born infection could account for cases of AIDS which have been discovered in hemophiliacs.

Seventy-five percent of the first 2500 cases of AIDS recorded by the Centers for Disease Control (CDC) in Atlanta, Georgia, have been either homosexual or bisexual men. The rapid spread of the "new" disease has resulted in a national "epidemic" of AIDS.

The first AIDS cases were reported by the CDC in June 1981. Early in the epidemic, AIDS was known as the GRID syndrome — an acronym for the Gay Related Immune Deficiency Syndrome. This term was quickly discarded when it was learned that some people with the disease were not gay. Many patients, their families, and gay rights advocates objected to the social stigma of the GRID syndrome, and to the scientific inaccuracy of the term.

More than three years after the start of the AIDS epidemic, the public is still confused and frightened by the inability of medical scientists to find the cause and cure of the illness. What is AIDS? Is it an infection? How contagious is it? Is it cancer? Where does the disease come from? Why can't it be cured?

Most medical experts insist that AIDS is a new disease which did not exist in America before 1979. Epidemiologists have claimed that sexual promiscuity among homosexual men, and drug abuse are "risk factors" in AIDS. These risk factors certainly existed in American society long before the epidemic of AIDS became apparent.

It is possible that small numbers of AIDS cases occurring in widely scattered areas of the country might have gone undetected for decades before the AIDS epidemic officially erupted in 1981. Up until the last few years, most homosexual men were still "in the closet," and very few men were openly "gay." It would have been most difficult for epidemiologists to tie in homosexuality to the epidemic of AIDS, simply because most gay men in the 1960s and 1970s were fearful of the social and legal consequences of publicly admitting their homosexuality.

Even today, homosexuality is taboo in Haitian society. For that reason, it has been difficult for American epidemiologists to uncover a history of homosexual activity in Haitian men with AIDS, because of the Haitian social stigma associated with homosexuality.

Nevertheless, it may be significant that the AIDS epidemic was initially recognized when physicians began to associate openly gay young men with unusual diseases, such as a heretofore unusual form of cancer known as Kaposi's sarcoma, and Pneumocystis pneumonia, a rare lung disease caused by a parasite.

Most scientists have now assumed that a sexually transmissible infectious agent is being passed from person-to-person in homosexual acts between promiscuous men. This "agent," believed to be a virus, is thought to cause AIDS. There is no evidence to indicate that homosexuality *per se* predisposes to AIDS because lesbians have not become ill with AIDS.

Most gay men with AIDS are *not* dying from some "unknown" disease. They are dying from "specific" types of cancer, and from well-recognized infectious diseases which have been studied for decades. Nevertheless, male homosexuals are considered to be responsible for the AIDS epidemic in America.

The word epidemic strikes fear in the minds of many. It is surprising that the world "epidemic" has not been used to describe the 440,000 Americans who die yearly of cancer. So far, the total number of deaths from AIDS has been far fewer than the staggering number of cancer deaths per year in America.

The existence of AIDS should not come as a surprise to epidemiologists who have always been aware that certain well-defined racial, cultural, and social groups often have unique statistics for certain infectious diseases as well as for certain types of cancer. In addition, sexual activity, sexual promiscuity, and celibacy have always altered the cancer rates in certain groups of people.

Therefore, it follows that the newly recognized homosexual community would also be affected by certain diseases unique to its members. However, because the infectivity of a sexually transmitted microbe does not depend on the sexual preference of its host, it is understandable why AIDS is now affecting other "groups" besides male homosexuals.

This book has been written to provide greater understanding of AIDS and its possible relationship to other diseases, such as cancer. Some of the ideas in this book may be controversial, and likely to be at odds with current scientific thought and opinion about AIDS.

Nevertheless, in view of the scientific ignorance regarding the cause and cure of AIDS, it is imperative that new ideas and concepts about AIDS be developed to halt the continuing spread of this epidemic.

This book provides evidence to show that the most probable cause of AIDS is a bacterial infectious agent. This conclusion is based on personal observations of bacteria in both living and fatal cases of AIDS, as well as the published findings of other research scientists which indicate that bacteria may be causative agents in cancer.

The idea that bacteria are the cause of AIDS is controversial. Most scientists believe that the causative agent in AIDS is a "virus," rather than a bacterium.

Much of what I have learned about bacteria in AIDS has come not from medical textbooks and journals, but from microscopic examinations of diseased tissue in AIDS. For this reason, I have come to some conclusions about the cause of AIDS (and cancer) which are very different from the views held by most of my colleagues in medicine and science.

This book is an opportunity for me to share this knowledge with people who are interested in new insights into the nature, origin, and cause of AIDS.

1 AIDS: The Acquired Immune Deficiency Syndrome

All seriously ill AIDS patients have one factor in common. By means of blood testing, all patients have weakened immune systems. One of the ways that a healthy immune system keeps the body well is by helping to ward off microbes that cause disease. Most AIDS patients have been well before "acquiring" the syndrome.

What is a syndrome? Ordinarily, doctors speak of diseases. Many diseases have a specific cause and well-defined physical signs and symptoms that enable doctors to diagnose these illnesses. But a syndrome often has some signs and symptoms that appear quite unrelated and lumped together in a mysterious fashion. For instance, some people with AIDS may have one or more "opportunistic infections," each produced by a different microbe. Other AIDS patients have cancer tumors, particularly a previously rare form of cancer known as Kaposi's sarcoma. Some people with AIDS have both infection and cancer. Because one or more of these diseases commonly occur in AIDS, the signs and symptoms produced by these different diseases can vary tremendously in persons with AIDS.

Some sexually active but otherwise healthy homosexual men have been found to be immunologically deficient.

Scientists are working hard to discover an infectious agent which might cause this immunodepression in AIDS. When this agent is discovered, the AIDS syndrome will then be known as a "specific" disease.

At present, there is no specific laboratory test to detect AIDS. Cancer patients receiving chemotherapy, and patients with hepatitis, infectious mononucleosis, and certain other diseases may show immunosuppression similar to AIDS patients.

AIDS is diagnosed with certainty if opportunistic infection and/or Kaposi's sarcoma appear in "high risk" patients. According to the criteria established by the Centers for Disease Control (CDC), AIDS cannot be diagnosed in patients with Kaposi's sarcoma who are over the age of sixty, or in patients who have been on immunosuppressive drugs for the treatment of cancer or other diseases.

The most common signs and symptoms that suggest a possible diagnosis of AIDS are:

1) swollen lymph glands ("nodes") for over six months duration
2) fatigue
3) fevers and night sweats
4) weight loss
5) diarrhea

Even though some or all of these symptoms may be present in homosexual or bisexual men, in most instances, AIDS with Kaposi's sarcoma and/or opportunistic infections *do not develop*. In May 1982, the CDC reviewed the data on 57 cases of gay or bisexual men with enlarged lymph nodes (lymphadenopathy). Many complained of fatigue, fever, and night sweats. Others had weight loss, and enlarged livers and spleens. Most of them had had venereal diseases, and drug use was common. Only *one* patient developed Kaposi's sarcoma during the period of observation.

In 1983, Donald Abrams, a physician at the University of California Cancer Research Institute in San Francisco, reported a study of 100 gay men with chronic enlargement of the lymph nodes. Although many of these men showed the same clinical and immunologic abnormalities as known AIDS patients, *none* developed Kaposi's sarcoma or opportunistic infection during a more than one-year period of observation. Although the men had received counseling on lifestyle changes and drug abuse, and had altered some of these factors, there was no improvement of the immune deficiency. Abrams hopes to determine if there is a link between the enlargement of the lymph glands and the unknown agent of AIDS. He also hopes to establish whether or not the gland abnormalities precede the onset of cancer and opportunistic infection.

The most common specific diseases which can develop in AIDS are cancer (particularly Kaposi's sarcoma and lymphoma) and parasitic Pneumocystis pneumonia. With the development of these serious and life-threatening diseases, the AIDS patient has a "specific" diagnosis *in addition to AIDS*. The onset of these diseases is further proof of the increased failing of the immune system.

Statistics for the sexual orientation of AIDS patients in 1983 were revealing. Male homosexuals, or bisexuals, comprised 75% of the cases (down from 94% in 1981). The remaining cases were male heterosexuals (15%), unknown sexual orientation (5%), and female heterosexuals (5%).

Groups of persons considered "at risk" in America for the development of AIDS include:

1) male homosexuals

2) intravenous drug abusers

3) Haitian refugees

4) hemophiliacs

5) infants receiving blood transfusions

6) female sexual partners of males with AIDS

7) male prison inmates

8) female prostitutes

The medical treatment for AIDS has been unusually difficult due to serious viral, bacterial, fungal, yeast, and parasitic infections which may develop in these immunodepressed patients. The development of cancer in a third of the AIDS cases has further complicated the treatment of these patients.

The epidemic of AIDS can only be well understood by studying the individual diseases, particularly Kaposi's sarcoma, and Pneumocystis pneumonia, which affect most of the seriously ill patients with AIDS.

By closely examining these diseases, we shall see that they are not "new" diseases. Kaposi's sarcoma has been endemic for many decades in central Africa and has affected thousands of black Africans. Pneumocystis pneumonia has already occurred in epidemic form in European babies, as well as in "mini-epidemics" in children's cancer wards in American hospitals.

References

CDC: *Persistent, generalized lymphadenopathy among homosexual males. MMWR 31:249-250, 1982.*

Abrams DI: *Lymphadenopathy but no apparent link to AIDS. Presented at the American Society of Clinical Oncology, 19th Annual Meeting, San Diego, California, 1983.*

2 "Gay" Kaposi's Sarcoma

In January 1979, a 44 year-old gay man noticed a red bump on the skin of his leg. He wondered if he could have bruised it, but the area wasn't painful, and he couldn't recall any injury. He assumed it would disappear as most red skin spots usually do.

By summer, he had become frightened. New spots had appeared on his arms, chest, back, and face. He finally consulted a doctor, who removed one of the red spots for a microscopic biopsy test. The pathologist diagnosed Kaposi's sarcoma, a rare form of cancer. He was referred to the Memorial Sloan-Kettering Cancer Center in New York City for further testing.

What was causing these tumors? He had always been fairly healthy. Several times he had come down with syphilis and gonorrhea, and he also had some prostate gland trouble, but basically he felt well. Nevertheless, the doctors were worried about the cancerous skin tumors, and he consented to chemotherapy.

By Christmas, he was experiencing frequent fevers and was admitted to Memorial Hospital in March 1980. New purple growths had appeared inside his mouth. His rectal area had ulcerated, due to a severe herpes virus infection. To make matters worse, he developed diarrhea caused by

9

intestinal parasites. He was given special antibiotics and prednisone, a form of cortisone.

He left the hospital, but was soon rehospitalized with a blockage of an artery behind his eye. The fever continued, along with the rectal ulcerations and diarrhea. New skin lesions of Kaposi's sarcoma now covered more than half his body. He was given more antibiotics, but despite treatment, he died with overwhelming infection in June 1980.

His family allowed an autopsy. Cancer tumors of Kaposi's sarcoma were discovered in the liver, stomach, lung, testes, spleen, and colon. The pathologist also detected a "cytomegalic" virus infection of the liver, lungs, pancreas, adrenal glands, urinary bladder, and colon.

One month earlier, another young gay man had also died of Kaposi's sarcoma at the New York Hospital. He had become extremely fatigued in July 1979. By fall, doctors discovered swollen glands in his neck and a biopsy test showed Kaposi's sarcoma tumors within the glands. He became dangerously ill with inflammation of the lungs, blood infections, and continuing fever. This patient died in May 1980. No autopsy was permitted.

Peculiarly, in January 1979, another 40 year-old homosexual man from New York City noticed a purplish bump on the roof of his mouth. By spring he was losing weight, and new purple and red spots were appearing on his skin. By summer, some of his lymph glands had enlarged and a biopsy test taken at Memorial Hospital showed Kaposi's sarcoma.

This patient had never had any serious illness. He had had syphilis and gonorrhea ten years earlier, and a bout with intestinal parasites four years earlier, but otherwise he felt fine. However, the doctors were alarmed about the increasing numbers of Kaposi's sarcoma skin lesions. He was treated unsuccessfully with cancer chemotherapy. In April 1980, he was started on a new drug regimen consisting of ten different immunosuppressive, anti-cancer drugs.

The skin lesions of Kaposi's sarcoma still did not change.

In July 1980 he entered Memorial Hospital with fever, diarrhea, and rectal pain. A variety of different infections were found, including a "Candida" yeast infection of the mouth, a herpes virus infection of the rectal area, and intestinal parasites. He suffered a stroke in October and died in December 1980.

At the autopsy, Kaposi's sarcoma and cytomegalic virus infection were found in some internal organs. The stroke had been caused by a rare parasitic infection called "toxoplasmosis."

The internal medicine doctors, the infectious disease experts, the cancer doctors (oncologists), the dermatologists, and the pathologists were perplexed. They were all seeing a disease they hadn't read about in medical textbooks and journals. But the disease was obviously a deadly one, and a disease they were powerless to stop.

In April 1981, Alvin Friedman-Kien, a dermatologist at New York University Medical Center, examined a young homosexual man thought to have a lymphoma (a form of lymph gland cancer). The purplish spots on the man's legs appeared quite unusual. Although the dermatologist was suspicious that the skin lesions might be Kaposi's sarcoma, he had never seen the disease in such a *young* person. The skin biopsy confirmed Friedman-Kien's suspicion.

Within a week, the dermatologist made another amazing discovery. A second gay man with Kaposi's sarcoma appeared in his skin clinic. The curious Friedman-Kien decided to make some phone calls around the city. He contacted colleagues at Memorial Hospital, who confirmed that they too had seen several cases of Kaposi's sarcoma in young men, some of whom had died terribly with severe and horrific infections.

Another phone call was made to Marcus Conant, a dermatologist at the University of California in San Francisco. Another of Friedman-Kien's suspicions was confirmed. Yes, Conant had recently seen several cases of Kaposi's sarcoma in young men living in the Bay area.

In an attempt to alert the medical community, Friedman-Kien reported the unusual and frightening outbreak of Kaposi's sarcoma cases in young gay men to the CDC in Atlanta.

On June 5, 1981, the CDC published its first bulletin concerning a rare and serious form of pneumonia called *Pneumocystis carinii* pneumonia which was occurring in young homosexual men in Los Angeles.

But the first alert of a serious epidemic of Kaposi's sarcoma in gay men was related by Friedman-Kien on June 26, 1981. A group of about one hundred gay and lesbian physicians was attending an historic symposium entitled "Medical Aspects of Sexual Orientation" held at the San Francisco Medical Society. The meeting, sponsored by the Bay Area Physicians for Human Rights, was the first national gathering of gay physicians ever held. The Symposium was taking place during Gay Pride weekend. A gay and lesbian parade takes place each June in San Francisco and attracts millions of spectators.

Friedman-Kien's symposium report on Kaposi's sarcoma in gay men in New York City was ominous. The disease was new, aggressive, often lethal, and was occurring in unprecedented numbers. The men were all highly active sexually. Most had medical histories of sexually transmitted diseases, and all used prescription and recreational drugs. The aggressive nature of Kaposi's sarcoma in gay men was similar to the type of Kaposi's sarcoma seen in Africa. All these gay patients were immunodepressed. Friedman-Kien, and his colleagues (*et al*), later commented on the gay lifestyle and its possible relationship to Kaposi's sarcoma, in a paper subsequently published in *The Annals of Internal Medicine*.

"The recent appearance of this disease may be associated with the changes that have occurred in the lifestyle of homosexual men living in large urban centers. There has been a marked increase in gay bathhouses, bars, and meeting places where multiple, anonymous sexual encounters occur. This has been reflected in a marked increase in the incidence of sexually transmitted diseases: not only syphilis and gonorrhea but also amebiasis, giardiasis, Epstein-Barr virus, and cytomegalovirus infections. Use of multiple recreational drugs, especially the inhalation of amyl and butyl nitrite, available through nonprescription sources, is also an important aspect of this changing lifestyle."

On July 3, 1981, the CDC published a second report entitled "Kaposi's sarcoma and Pneumocystis pneumonia among homosexual men, New York and California." Twenty six homosexual men were reported with Kaposi's sarcoma. Eight patients had already died. In the follow-up report by the CDC (August 28, 1981), seventy additional cases of Kaposi's sarcoma and Pneumocystis pneumonia were recorded.

Based on these reports, the National Cancer Institute and the CDC sponsored a workshop on Kaposi's sarcoma on September 15, 1981, at the National Institute of Health in Bethesda, Maryland. At that time, 55 cases of Kaposi's sarcoma, 49 cases of Pneumocystis pneumonia, and 11 cases of both diseases had been reported. All of these cases were men, — 94% of whom were homosexual or bisexual. Eighty percent of the patients were between 25 and 45 years of age.

Infectious disease experts concluded that "at present, cytomegalovirus is the leading candidate for an etiologic role in Kaposi's sarcoma; recommendations for future studies are heavily oriented toward this virus. While evidence for a relationship between cytomegalovirus and Kaposi's sarcoma has been steadily mounting, there are some as yet unresolved discrepancies. It is essential, therefore, to keep an open mind and to look for other viruses that might be associated with the tumor."

The epidemic had begun. Within three years the epidemic of AIDS was to prove far more devastating than the Legionnaires' disease epidemic which had occurred, in America, in 1976. Less than six months after the onset of that epidemic, a causative bacterium was discovered, much to the amazement of all the medical and scientific experts who had been looking for a suspected virus. No one had seen the bacterium before, but it was perfectly capable of producing a serious epidemic.

But bacteria couldn't possibly be causing Kaposi's sarcoma. "Classic" Kaposi's sarcoma had been around for over a century. There was never the slightest indication that it was contagious or even infectious. At least, not until the epidemic of AIDS and the marked rise in the number of cases of "Gay" cancer in promiscuous homosexual men.

References

Urmacher C, Myskowski P, Ochoa M, *et al: Outbreak of Kaposi's sarcoma with cytomegalovirus infection in young homosexual men. Amer J Med 72:569-575, 1982.*

CDC: *Pneumocystis pneumonia — Los Angeles. MMWR 30: 250-252, 1981.*

Friedman-Kien AE: *Kaposi's sarcoma. Presented at a symposium entitled Medical Aspects in Sexual Orientation, Bay Area Physicians for Human Rights, San Francisco, California, June 26-27, 1981.*

Friedman-Kien AE, Laubenstein L, Rubinstein P, *et al: Disseminated Kaposi's sarcoma in homosexual men. Ann Intern Med 96:693-704, 1982.*

CDC: *Kaposi's sarcoma and Pneumocystis pneumonia among homosexual men — New York City and California. MMWR 30:305-307, 1981.*

CDC: *Follow-up on Kaposi's sarcoma and Pneumocystis pneumonia. MMWR 30:409-410, 1981.*

DeWys WD, Curran J, Henle W, *et al: Workshop on Kaposi's sarcoma: Meeting report. Cancer Treat Rep 66:1387-1390, 1982.*

3 "Classic" Kaposi's Sarcoma

The two pathologists at the George Washington School of Medicine in Washington, D.C., were amazed. Roger Choisser and Elizabeth Ramsey had just finished studying the autopsy of a 30 year-old policeman who had died of a very rare, blood-filled cancer tumor which had formed inside his heart. Six weeks earlier, the same pathologists had autopsied another young man, 26 years of age, who had died after the rupture of a similar blood-filled tumor which had also formed inside his heart.

Both young men had been strong and vigorous until two months before their deaths. Both had been hospitalized with enlarged hearts, shortness of breath, and extreme weakness. Two months before he died, the first man had had a "cold" and bronchitis. The other man had had the "flu." His symptoms of weakness, night sweats, and fever continued until his death.

The pathologists found large tumors of Kaposi's sarcoma within the right auricular area of the heart of both men. Most patients with Kaposi's sarcoma have blood tumors of the skin. But, strangely, these men had none. The pathologists were surprised at the comparative youth of the men and the fact that both were native-born Americans. The rapidly fatal course of the disease was also highly unusual.

Today, doctors would want to know if these patients were

"straight" or "gay," married or single, promiscuous or monogamous. Did they take illegal drugs? Did they know each other socially?

But these questions were hardly appropriate when these two young men died. *The year was 1939.* Forty years before the AIDS epidemic was uncovered.

Before the onset of AIDS in America, Kaposi's sarcoma was a very rare disease. Annual cancer statistics indicated that three people out of one million might develop Kaposi's sarcoma. Most physicians had never seen a case, and the disease was studied primarily by pathologists and dermatologists.

The development of Kaposi's sarcoma and other forms of cancer in AIDS patients is one of the most frightening aspects of the new epidemic. Kaposi's sarcoma may appear as one or more reddish patches or lumps (nodules) on the skin. Similar tumors may appear within the internal organs, especially the intestines, and within the lymph nodes. Hemorrhage of such blood-filled tumors frequently causes death.

The diagnosis of Kaposi's sarcoma is made by removing all or part of the tumor and by submitting the biopsy tissue to the pathologist for examination. The biopsy specimen is processed and cut thinly into "sections" which are then stained and prepared for microscopic examination and diagnosis by the pathologist.

Tumors of Kaposi's sarcoma are composed of distinctive cancer cells called "spindle cells." The tumors also contain large numbers of newly-formed capillary blood vessels, as well as new vascular "slits" filled with red blood cells. The purple and red color of Kaposi's sarcoma skin tumors is due to the abnormal number of new blood-filled vessels and spaces within the tumor.

Until 1950, there were only about 600 cases of Kaposi's sarcoma recorded in the world medical literature. However, the supposed rarity of the disease, before AIDS, may have been because many cases were not recorded in cancer registries or reported in medical journals.

Samuel Bluefarb, a dermatologist, wrote in his book "Kaposi's Sarcoma" (1957), that "in many large cities, Kaposi's sarcoma is not reported unless the patient exhibits unusual manifestations of the disease."

Bluefarb's view was reiterated in 1973, by three dermatologists in New York City, who recorded one hundred people from that area with biopsy-proven skin lesions of Kaposi's sarcoma. The 100 patients in this one city ranged in age from 40 to 89 years. Seventy-eight were men. Fifty three were Jewish, and eighteen were Italian. Follow-up information on fifty six patients revealed that no one had died of Kaposi's sarcoma.

The study concluded that "this is apparently the largest series of patients with Kaposi's sarcoma ever reported in the western world. The large amount of material in this study, the relative ease with which it was collected, and the follow-up information obtained thus far suggest that many cases of Kaposi's sarcoma are not referred to large medical centers, and are not listed in tumor registries, but are diagnosed and treated in the community. *Thus, the true incidence and prevalence of Kaposi's sarcoma is probably several times that estimated in the literature.*" (Author's italics). The researchers pointed out that "the great majority of patients with Kaposi's sarcoma follow a benign course and are adequately diagnosed and treated in the office of a dermatologist."

Until the end of the 1970s little attention was paid to Kaposi's sarcoma in America because the disease was uncommon and rarely caused death. Only in certain parts of Africa was the incidence of Kaposi's sarcoma known to be two hundred times more common, and to be a frequently fatal disease, particularly in young men and children.

However, by 1979, it was becoming increasingly clear

that Kaposi's sarcoma could develop and pose a serious threat to life in people who had undergone kidney transplantation. These patients were given immunosuppressive drugs, in order to protect the newly transplanted kidney. Without these drugs, a patient's immune system would attempt to reject the transplanted kidney.

In patients who receive organ transplants, the chances of developing Kaposi's sarcoma were found to be 400 to 500 times greater than normal. Andrew Harwood, *et al* (1979), from Toronto, Canada, concluded that "the increased incidence of Kaposi's sarcoma in renal transplant recipients suggests that immunosuppression may be important in the development of the disease." When immunosuppressive drugs were discontinued, the tumors of Kaposi's sarcoma often diminished in size or disappeared.

Kaposi's sarcoma has always been a peculiar form of cancer. Some tumors of Kaposi's sarcoma may persist for decades, and have also been known to vanish as mysteriously as they appeared. Unlike regular cancer tumors that develop at one particular site, and then spread (metastasize) to other areas of the body, Kaposi's sarcoma may occur as multiple tumors from the very onset of the disease.

There has always been controversy as to whether Kaposi's sarcoma is a malignant or a benign form of cancer. Some investigators have even suggested that Kaposi's sarcoma is not cancer, but rather an infection, perhaps due to a virus. Some pathologists even question whether Kaposi's sarcoma is a "true" sarcoma.

Where do the malignant "spindle cells" of Kaposi's sarcoma tumors come from? Do the cancerous "spindle cells" originate from blood vessel cells, connective tissue cells, reticuloendothelial cells, or nerve cells? Scientists simply do not know. Because the cancer cell type is not known, Kaposi's sarcoma may not even be a "sarcoma" at all.

One of the most distressing features of Kaposi's sarcoma is that more than one-third of the people with this form of cancer will eventually develop *another* kind of cancer, usually of the leukemic or lymph gland (lymphoma) type.

Kaposi's sarcoma patients are twenty times as likely to get these kinds of cancer!

Kaposi's sarcoma was first reported by Moriz Kaposi in 1872. Between 1868 and 1871, Kaposi studied five patients with these tumors. All were men between the ages of 40 and 68 who had come to his dermatology clinic in Vienna, Austria.

Kaposi described the tumors as "nodules the size of shot, peas, or hazelnuts, and brown-red to blue-red in color, which develop in the skin without a known general or local cause. They ordinarily appear first on the sole of the foot and the instep, and not long afterwards, also on the hands. *The disease is rapidly lethal, within two to three years.*"

Today, most physicians consider "classic" Kaposi's sarcoma as one of the least life-threatening forms of cancer. However, as quoted, this was *not* Kaposi's original conception of the disease, which he declared to be "rapidly lethal."

Kaposi was also aware that Kaposi's sarcoma tumors could also be found *inside* the body. One century later, these rare skin tumors, bearing Kaposi's name, would be a dreaded sign in the diagnosis of AIDS in homosexual men.

Moriz Kaposi was born in 1837, in Kaposvar, a small country town on the river Kapos, in southern Hungary. Both parents were Jewish and he was named Moriz Kohn, at birth. After graduating from medical school at the University of Vienna, he worked as a surgeon and obstetrician. He became avidly interested in the study of skin diseases and eventually joined the internationally famous dermatology clinic, in Vienna, headed by Professor von Hebra. In 1869, still under the name Kohn, he married Professor Hebra's daughter.

Kaposi formally changed his name from Kohn to Kaposi in 1871. According to Karl Holubar and Jozsef Frankl

(1981), Kaposi's reason was that "Kohn is a name carried by hundreds of people of various classes and of different professions; mistakes are constantly and increasingly made about persons carrying the same name. At Vienna University alone, there were concurrently five doctors with a similar surname. Kaposi explicitly stated that it was for these reasons alone that he wished to change his name in such a way that the name of his native city Kaposvar henceforth be celebrated in the form of an adjective, Kaposi. As regards pronunciation, the river Kapos, the town Kaposvar, and the name Kaposi all carry the accent on the first syllable and not, as frequently heard in Anglo-Saxon countries, on the second."

Stephen Rothman (1962), also gave instructions for the Hungarian pronunciation of Kaposi's acquired name. "It is probably a hopeless and useless endeavor to teach the correct pronunciation of the Hungarian name Kaposi to an English and French-speaking audience. Suffice it to say that the accent is on the first syllable as in all Hungarian words. The vowel 'a' is short and pronounced as in the English word 'wardrobe' and the vowel 'o' as in the word 'off.' The consonant 's' should be pronounced as 'sh' in English."

Kaposi became head of the Dermatology Department after Hebra's death in 1880. The closing years of the nineteenth century brought Kaposi international fame, and many honors for his scientific achievements. He was an excellent speaker, being fluent in Hungarian, German, French, and English. He died in 1902, at which time the Vienna School of Dermatology was the most highly regarded school in the scientific world.

More than a century after the discovery of the disease, the cause of Kaposi's sarcoma remains a mystery. However, one thing is new and certain. Kaposi's sarcoma is occurring in unprecedented numbers in homosexual men in New York City, San·Francisco, Los Angeles, and other American cities. For the first time in medical history a sexually transmitted microbe is thought to be a possible cause of this type of cancer.

Kaposi would have been surprised by the current idea that Kaposi's sarcoma might be infectious, or even contagious. At the time he discovered the disease (1872), microbes were not accepted as the cause of *any* infectious disease. Even after "acid-fast" tuberculosis mycobacteria were shown to be the cause of skin tuberculosis in 1882, Kaposi persisted in denying the existence of this kind of infection.

A century later, researchers would be finding "viruses" and "acid-fast bacteria" in tumors of Kaposi's sarcoma. But, like Kaposi, physicians would still be highly skeptical as to the significance of these microbes. Scientists would continue to search for the true and proven infectious agent that was causing the epidemic of AIDS.

References

Choisser RM, and Ramsey EM: *Angioreticuloendothelioma (Kaposi's disease) of the heart. Amer J Pathol 15: 155-177, 1939.*

Bluefarb SM: *Kaposi's Sarcoma. Charles C. Thomas, Springfield, Illinois, 1957.*

Brownstein MH, Sharpiro L, Skolnik P: *Kaposi's sarcoma in community practice. Arch Dermatol 107:137-138, 1973.*

Harwood AR, Osoba D, Hofstader SL, *et al: Kaposi's sarcoma in recipients of renal transplants. Amer J Med 67:759-765, 1979.*

Kaposi M: *Idiopathic multiple pigmented sarcoma of the skin. Ca, A Cancer Journal for Clinicians 32: 342-347, 1982. (Translated from the German and reprinted from Archiv fur Dermatologie und Syphilis 4:265-273, 1872).*

Haverkos HW, and Curran JW: *The current outbreak of Kaposi's sarcoma and opportunistic infections. Ca, A Cancer Journal for Clinicians 32:330-337, 1982.*

Holubar K, and Frank J: *Moriz (Kohn) Kaposi. Amer J Dermatopathol 3:349-354, 1981.*

Rothman S: *Some remarks on Moricz Kaposi and on the history of Kaposi's sarcoma. Acta Un Int Cancr 18:322-325, 1962.*

Weidenfeld DR: *Moritz Kaposi. In memoriam. Amer J Dermatopathol 3:355-358, 1981. (Translated from the German and reprinted from Wiener Medizinesche Presse 11:519-523, 1902).*

Braun M: *Moriz Kaposi M.D. Ca, A Cancer Journal for Clinicians 32:340-341, 1982.*

(*) Kaposi's name, Moriz/Moritz/Moricz, appears with various spellings in scientific literature.

4 African Kaposi's Sarcoma

During January 1980, while the reports of the first cases of Kaposi's sarcoma in young American homosexual men were filtering into the Centers for Disease Control (CDC) in Atlanta, Georgia, the second African "Symposium on Kaposi's Sarcoma" was taking place at Makerere College Medical School, in Kampala, Uganda. A similar group of medical experts had previously convened nineteen years earlier, in the same African city, to discuss Kaposi's sarcoma, an endemic and frequently fatal malignant disease common in Central Africa.

For some reason yet to be discovered, the tropical portion of the equatorial belt, extending from the Congo across East Africa, has the world's highest incidence of Kaposi's sarcoma. The countries most affected are Zaire, Rwanda and Burundi, Tanzania, French Equatorial Africa, Uganda, Zimbabwe, and Kenya.

One could only guess as to how long this epidemic number of cases of Kaposi's sarcoma had been occurring. Doctors caring for people in these third world countries have been preoccupied by the treatment of infectious and parasitic diseases. As a result, records and statistics of cancer incidence in Africa have simply not been available for study, until recent years.

The eastern, tropical portion of Zaire has the world's

highest incidence of Kaposi's sarcoma, with this form of cancer comprising 9% of all the malignant tumors in that nation. In Uganda, during the years 1964-1969, 359 cases were recorded, accounting for over 5% of all malignant tumors examined microscopically. Only cancer of the penis, and cancer of the liver, are more common tumors in Ugandan men. Across the border in Tanzania, Kaposi's sarcoma accounts for over 4% of tumors. Young men are affected *ten times* as often as women. The reason for this is unknown. It is very rare for more than one family member to acquire the disease. Among children with Kaposi's sarcoma, the male-female ratio is much lower, around 3 to 1.

Although the disease is common in black Africans, Kaposi's sarcoma is rarely observed in white Africans and Indians, even those living there for several generations. According to M. S. Hutt, a geographical pathologist from London, the incidence rates of Kaposi's sarcoma are much lower in West and South Africa, although they are still significantly higher than elsewhere in the world. North African countries are relatively unaffected by Kaposi's sarcoma. Some physicians at the conference thought that certain geographic areas with a high incidence of Kaposi's sarcoma corresponded to areas of heavy rainfall in Africa.

Some African men, especially those over the age of thirty, have Kaposi's sarcoma skin tumors confined primarily to the legs. This may result in severe swelling (edema) of the feet and ankles. When the tumors occur internally, the disease becomes more serious. Especially dangerous are blood tumors of the intestines which can rupture and cause death. Kaposi's sarcoma tumors may persist for as long as twenty five years, and some tumors may disappear without treatment. In this respect, some African cases resemble "classic" cases of Kaposi's sarcoma, occurring in elderly heterosexual American and European men.

One serious form of African Kaposi's sarcoma attacks young men *under* the age of 30. Internal tumors of Kaposi's sarcoma are common, and may be rapidly fatal. This type of

Kaposi's sarcoma is similar to that seen in young homosexual men with AIDS in America.

Another serious form of African Kaposi's sarcoma affects children. Death may occur within one year. Skin tumors of Kaposi's sarcoma are not present, but the lymph glands may enlarge tremendously. In the early stages of AIDS, some homosexual men may have similar enlargement of the glands, which may precede the onset of Kaposi's sarcoma and opportunistic infections.

It is only with the recent epidemic of AIDS and Kaposi's sarcoma that attention has been redirected to African Kaposi's sarcoma. In 1957 Samuel Bluefarb wrote in his classic monograph, "Kaposi's Sarcoma," that "Kaposi's sarcoma appears to be comparatively rare in the (American) Negro race." But Bluefarb did alert physicians to the relatively high incidence of Kaposi's sarcoma in black Africans.

At the 1980 African Symposium, a Tanzanian, J. Shaba asked: "What is the incidence of Kaposi's sarcoma among the American Negroes?"

C. L. Vogel, from the Comprehensive Cancer Center in Miami, Florida, responded: "Kaposi's sarcoma is a very rare tumor in the United States. Of interest, however, is the fact that since my return to the United States, I have seen only four cases of Kaposi's sarcoma and all the four patients were women. I would like very much to see some statistics on Kaposi's sarcoma from the United States, although I am not sure where they will come from since the tumor is so rare."

Gaetano Giraldo, a researcher from Memorial Sloan-Kettering Cancer Center in New York City, and a leading proponent of the cytomegalovirus theory of Kaposi's sarcoma, also agreed that "Kaposi's sarcoma is extremely rare in the United States."

One of the most distinctive and unusual microscopic findings in African tumors of Kaposi's sarcoma is the presence of red-stained (eosinophilic) "inclusion bodies" within the Kaposi's sarcoma tumor cells and within the surrounding cancerous tissue. The microscopic size of these round "inclusion bodies" varies from tiny, barely visible particles up to the size of red blood cells. F. D. Lee, a Ugandan pathologist, found these inclusions in the Kaposi's sarcoma tissue sections in 60% of his cases, and thought these particles might represent "degenerative changes." Lee believed that these inclusions in Kaposi's sarcoma were similar in appearance to "Russell bodies." William Russell was a Scottish pathologist who discovered round "bodies" in cancer tissue in 1890. Russell believed that these bodies were microbes which were the cause of cancer. We will discuss Russell's bodies again when we review the history of the "cancer microbe."

The actual nature of eosinophilic "inclusion bodies" in African Kaposi's sarcoma tumors is not known. Lee, like Russell, found similar bodies in other forms of cancer. But Lee also thought that the "inclusion bodies" might be *viral* in nature. This conjecture seems worthy of further study, particularly since the cytomegalovirus is currently being proposed as a likely cause of Kaposi's sarcoma.

During the symposium, Giraldo, the well-known researcher whose viral studies in Kaposi's sarcoma largely form the scientific evidence on which the viral theory of AIDS and Kaposi's sarcoma is based, was asked if he thought the "inclusion bodies" were significant, or suggestive of a "possible viral cause" of Kaposi's sarcoma. He responded: "I do not really think these are virus-related inclusion bodies. The morphology is somewhat different and in addition, we have done at the beginning of our study, large screening by electron microscopy of Kaposi's sarcoma and we have never seen any type of viral particles in the primary stages or viral related bodies. I do not believe these inclusion bodies are viral related."

Although other researchers have not reported eosinophilic "inclusion bodies" in American cases of Kaposi's sarcoma, Alan Cantwell and Jerry Lawson have shown tiny granular forms in Kaposi's sarcoma tumors occurring in both elderly men, and in young men with AIDS. These forms are similar in appearance to the inclusion bodies described and illustrated by Lee, and other pathologists, in African cases. Cantwell believes these granular forms are bacteria.

There is evidence that an increasing number of American AIDS cases, (with or without Kaposi's sarcoma), are suffering from opportunistic infection caused by an "acid-fast" mycobacterium called *Mycobacterium avium-intracellulare*. This so-called "atypical" acid-fast mycobacterium is closely related to the acid-fast mycobacterium, (*Mycobacterium tuberculosis*), that causes tuberculosis. As many as one-third of the Haitians in America with AIDS also have tuberculosis.

Closely allied to the finding of acid-fast bacteria in some AIDS patients, is the remarkable finding presented at the African Symposium which indicated that leprosy, (also known as Hansen's disease), often preceded the onset of Kaposi's sarcoma in African men. This is an important revelation, because leprosy is a bacterial infection *also* caused by acid-fast bacteria, (*Mycobacterium leprae*). This African finding indicates that acid-fast mycobacterial "opportunistic infection" might play an important role in the development of Kaposi's sarcoma in Blacks in Africa, just as mycobacteria do in some Gays and Haitians in America with AIDS.

The symposium dialog on this subject is revealing:

Charles Olweny from the Uganda Cancer Institute declared, "I have recently been impressed by the number of patients coming to the Uganda Cancer Institute from either Nyenga or Buluba Leprosarium. Is Kaposi's sarcoma sometimes mistaken for leprosy or do the diseases occur together in the same patient?"

H. Blenska of the Buluba Leprosarium, Uganda, responded, "Kaposi's sarcoma is astonishingly associated with both tuberculoid and lepromatous leprosy."

And, D. H. Novak of the Nyenga Hospital, Uganda,

added, "Our cases of Kaposi's sarcoma were usually patients who have undergone anti-leprosy treatment for many years and were cured of their leprosy."

These observations, never discussed in America, indicate that some black Africans have had pre-existing, or coexisting infection, with leprosy bacteria, prior to the development of Kaposi's sarcoma. Similarly, some Haitians have had tuberculosis due to acid-fast bacteria, and some gay men have had "atypical" tuberculosis due to "atypical" acid-fast bacteria. "African," "Haitian," and "Gay" Kaposi's sarcoma are *all* strikingly similar, in that the disease can be rapidly fatal, especially in younger men. Kaposi's sarcoma, largely confined to Central Africa, is also largely confined to coastal cities in America, such as New York City, San Francisco, Los Angeles, and Miami.

In reporting the proceedings of the African Symposium, Charles Olweny proclaimed the conference a success. Olweny regarded the various reports and presentations as a possible reflection of "the state of the art" on Kaposi's sarcoma in 1980. *No participant regarded Kaposi's sarcoma as a sexually transmitted disease.*

It is unlikely that any expert on Kaposi's sarcoma in 1980 could have predicted that future symposia on epidemic Kaposi's sarcoma would take place not in Africa, but rather in New York, San Francisco, Los Angeles, and other American cities where Kaposi's sarcoma in homosexual men would be one of the most dreaded diseases encountered in the new epidemic of AIDS.

References

Olweny CLM, Hutt MSR, Owor R (Eds): *Kaposi's Sarcoma, in Antibiotics Chemother: 29, S Karger, Basel, Switzerland, 1981. (2nd Kaposi's Sarcoma Symposium, Kampala, January 8-11, 1980).*

Hutt MSR: *The epidemiology of Kaposi's sarcoma, in Kaposi's Sarcoma, Antibiotics Chemother 29:3-8, 1981 (S Karger, Basel).*

Bluefarb SM: *Kaposi's Sarcoma, Charles C Thomas, Springfield, 1957, p 10.*

Slavin G, Cameron HM, Singh H: *Kaposi's sarcoma in mainland Tanzania: A report of 117 cases. Brit J Cancer 23: 349-357, 1969.*

Bhana D, Templeton HC, Master SP, *et al: Kaposi's sarcoma of lymph nodes. Brit J Cancer 24:464-470, 1970.*

Templeton AC, and Bhana D: *Prognosis in Kaposi's sarcoma. J Natl Cancer Inst 56:1301-1304, 1975.*

Lee FD: *A comparative study of Kaposi's sarcoma and granuloma pyogenicum in Uganda. J Clin Pathol 21:119-128, 1968.*

Russell W: *An address on a characteristic organism of cancer. Brit Med J 2:1356-1360, 1890.*

Giraldo G, Beth E, Kyalwazi SK: *Etiological implications on Kaposi's sarcoma, in Antibiotics Chemother 29: 12-32, 1981 (S Karger, Basel).*

Cantwell AR Jr: *Bacteriologic investigation and histologic observations of variably acid-fast bacteria in three cases of cutaneous Kaposi's sarcoma. Growth 45:79-89, 1981.*

Cantwell AR Jr, Lawson JW: *Necroscopic findings of pleomorphic, variably acid-fast bacteria in a fatal case of Kaposi's sarcoma. J Dermatol Surg Oncol 7:923-930, 1981.*

Cantwell AR Jr: *Variably acid-fast bacteria in vivo in a case of reactive lymph node hyperplasia occurring in a young male homosexual. Growth 46:331-336, 1982.*

Olweny CLM, Blenska H, Novak DH, *et al: Discussions of clinical features, in Antibiotic Chemother 29:68-69, 1981 (S Karger, Basel).*

Zakowski P, Fligiel S, Berlin GW, *et al: Disseminated Mycobacterium avium-intracellulare infection in homosexual men dying of acquired immunodeficiency. JAMA 248:2980-2982, 1982.*

5 Pneumocystis carinii Pneumonia

Ron was 44 years-old when he entered a San Francisco hospital in April, 1981. He had been sick for months with fever and diarrhea. His doctor had found intestinal parasites and had given him the proper medication. But Ron still was not improving. He couldn't understand why he felt so poorly. He had always been healthy except for bouts of hepatitis and syphilis years before. It was strange. The doctors at the hospital seemed to place great importance on the fact that he was gay. Ron couldn't understand why. After all, that was no big deal in San Francisco.

The first routine chest X-ray examination was normal, but three days later he began to have trouble breathing, along with an annoying cough. A second X-ray picture showed "infiltrates" of pneumonia. His breathing and cough worsened. Stephen Follansbee, and the other doctors, were worried. Five days later, a piece of his lung tissue was removed for biopsy testing. The pathologist was amazed to discover that the lung tissue was severely infected with a "protozoan parasite" called *Pneumocystis carinii.*

Ron was given an antibotic drug called trimethoprim to kill the parasites. He improved. Three weeks later he left the hospital, relieved that at least no evidence of intestinal parasites was found.

He saw the doctors regularly for the constant complaint

of tiredness. They always looked at the white patches inside his mouth, which they said were caused by a chronic yeast infection due to *Candida albicans*. It was peculiar. He was given medication to kill the yeast germs, but it never worked. By mid-August, the fever, the cough, and the breathing trouble returned. Two weeks later, Ron was back in the hospital.

Another lung biopsy test showed Pneumocystis parasites again. Though given the same antibiotic, he worsened. A new experimental drug was ordered from the CDC in Atlanta. The drug seemed to work, but now he needed a mechanical respirator to breathe. He stabilized for a while. No Pneumocystis parasites were found in the third lung biopsy test. After twelve days the new drug was discontinued. Five days later, a fourth lung biopsy again showed the dreaded parasite.

The experimental drug was restarted. Ron's special blood test showed a severely depressed immunologic state, and his lungs continued to weaken. His heart was showing electrocardiographic signs of irritability and his blood pressure was dropping. After thirty one days in the hospital, Ron died.

At the autopsy, his lungs showed microscopic evidence of "chronic interstitial pneumonitis." Not one, but *two* infectious agents had racked his lungs. The pathologist saw the parasite *Pneumocystis carinii*, which had plagued Ron for months. But there were also pathologic changes in the lung tissue caused by a virus called cytomegalovirus. For some unknown reason, Pneumocystis parasites and cytomegalovirus are often found together in diseased lungs. The combination can be deadly.

By June 1981, the first cases of opportunistic infection with *Pneumocystis carinii* in gay men were reported by the CDC. Until 1955, human infection with Pneumocystis was unknown in the United States. There simply were no recorded cases. What did medical science know about Pneumocystis? And why were healthy young gay men dying of Pneumocystis pneumonia?

Carlos Chagas, a microbiologist in Rio de Janiero, Brazil, first observed the parasite *Pneumocystis carinii* in 1909, in the lungs of guinea pigs. Chagas was experimenting with guinea pigs which he had deliberately infected with another kind of parasite, called the "trypanosome" parasite. When the guinea pigs were sacrificed and their lung tissue examined microscopically, Chagas saw the Pneumocystis parasite. Chagas assumed, (incorrectly), the Pneumocystis parasites were the trypanosome parasites which he had injected into the animals. The Brazilian scientist later became world famous for his discovery of "South American trypanosomiasis," (later called "Chagas' disease"), a protozoal parasitic disease which is transmitted by insects to humans.

A. Carini, another Brazilian microbiologist, also began to study the Pneumocystis parasite in 1910 in the lungs of rats experimentally infected with trypanosomes. Carini, like his colleague Chagas, also mistook Pneumocystis parasites for trypanosomes.

In 1912, Pneumocystis parasites were found in the lungs of sewer rats, in Paris. The discovery was made by Monsieur and Madame Delanoe, microbiologists at the Pasteur Institute. The Delanoes quickly realized that the parasite was unrelated to trypanosome infection because Parisian rats did not have the disease.

Out of scientific respect for Carini, who had diligently studied the parasite in Brazil, the Delanoes named the bihemispheric parasite *Pneumocystis carinii* in his honor. Subsequently, the Brazilian scientists and other microbiologists found the parasite in the lungs of a wide variety of animals including dogs, rabbits, and monkeys.

Chagas, in 1911, was the first to see the Pneumocystis parasite in the lungs of a human being. The patient was a Brazilian man who had died of South American trypanosomiasis. At the time of this discovery, Chagas was still assuming wrongly that the Pneumocystis parasites were the trypanosomal parasites which had killed the man. However, medical historians will undoubtedly forgive Chagas for this minor misinterpretation. It would be over thirty years before anyone in the entire scientific world would again see and recognize *Pneumocystis carinii* in the lungs of another human being!

Pneumocystis carinii was next encountered, in 1942, in the Netherlands. Mademoiselle van der Meer, and Monsieur Brug, microbiologists at the Institute of Tropical Hygiene, in Amsterdam, found the parasite in the lungs of two infants, and in a young man. According to their report, the parasite was apparently producing no lung disease. Understandably, this report provoked little scientific interest until a decade later when the mystery of a deadly epidemic of pneumonia was being unraveled.

Little or no attention would have been paid to *Pneumocystis carinii* were it not for cases of a peculiar type of sometimes fatal pneumonia occurring in children, in Europe. The first few recognized cases of "interstitial pneumonia" were reported in German infants in the late 1930s. During the 1940s, and into the 1950s, the disease was common in central Europe. Over 700 cases were reported in Switzerland between 1941 and 1948. Hamburg, Germany had 191 cases between 1950 and 1954. Czechoslovakia reported 196 cases in 1954. A children's hospital, in Yugoslavia, recorded 45 cases in 1954. Thirty four cases were identified, as far away as Finland, in northern Europe.

The lung disease usually struck infants during the first year of life, especially those prematurely born. The infants became restless, languid, and took feedings poorly. The breathing rate increased, alerting doctors to the possibility of lung disease. Strangely, the children coughed little or not at all. Fever was unusual. As the lungs become more damaged, breathing became more rapid, and labored. The children's skin paled. Frightening bluish tinges of cyanosis appeared around the mouth and eyes. The children were given oxygen. The lucky infants recovered slowly, with good nursing care. The unfortunate ones died within a few days to a few weeks.

When the X-ray pictures of the chest were held up to the light, the infected lungs had a distinctive "ground-glass" appearance. During epidemics, European radiologists became familiar with these "glassy" lungs. This X-ray sign was often helpful in the diagnosis of "infantile pneumonitis." A similar descriptive phrase would be used, three decades later, by Gordon Gamsu, and other San Francisco radiologists, to describe the ground-glass appearance of the lungs of homosexual men dying of AIDS, and the same kind of parasitic pneumonia.

At post-mortem examinations, pathologists noted almost complete airlessness in the children's lungs. The normal lung tissue and air passageways were smothered and infiltrated by large numbers of inflammatory cells, which some European pathologists called "mononuclear cells." American pathologists later called them "plasma cells" and "lymphocytes."

The credit for the discovery that *Pneumocystis carinii* was the actual cause of epidemic infantile interstitial pneumonia must go to J. Vanek, Professor of Pathology, at the Medical School in Plzen, Czechoslovakia. In 1951, he began to publish a series of scientific papers which clearly showed parasites in the lungs of every infant.

Vanek also made another extremely interesting observation in 1952. He reported a case of a sixty year-old woman with lymph gland cancer, (Hodgkin's disease), who also had both *Pneumocystis carinii* and cytomegalovirus infection of the lung. Three decades later, the occurrence of these three different diseases (cancer, Pneumocystis pneumonia, and cytomegalovirus infection), in young American homosexuals, would comprise one of the most frightening aspects of the AIDS epidemic. Over the next four years, (1951-1955), over sixty confirmatory reports in the Czechoslovakian, German, Austrian, and French medical literature attested to the correctness of Vanek's discovery.

In 1953, a report in *Pediatrics* by William Deamer and Hans Zollinger, from the Institute of Pathology at the University of Zurich in Switzerland, alerted American doctors to the epidemic of infantile "plasma cell pneumonia" in Europe. The pediatrician, and the pathologist, wrote: "it is remarkable that a disease so frequently seen and well-known in Switzerland, and several other European countries, should remain unnoticed in the United States. So that the reader may decide the latter point for himself, as well as to be alerted to the possible future occurrence of the illness, this report has been written." The investigators were aware of published reports by Vanek, and others, proclaiming *Pneumocystis carinii* as the cause of infantile "plasma cell pneumonia." Nevertheless Deamer and Zollinger regarded the parasites as "secondary invaders" of diseased tissue. Instead, they concluded that "the most commonly held opinion, in which the authors concur, is that the disease is infectious and probably of viral origin, but as yet there has been no convincing demonstration of the etiologic agent."

Deamer and Zollinger were prophetic in their 1953 report. In that same year the first American, a 7 week-old white baby boy, died in a Wisconsin hospital after a month-long respiratory infection. This case was reported in 1955, by a group of four pathologists and pediatricians, as "interstitial plasma cell pneumonia." No mention was made of the numerous reports from Europe indicating that *Pneumocystis carinii* was commonly found in the lungs of fatal cases of "interstitial pneumonia." The investigators simply reiterated the view that "the failure to culture organisms from any case suggests that the infectious agent may be a virus."

In 1956, a report entitled "Pneumocystis infection and cytomegaly of the lungs in the newborn and adult," by H. Hamperl, a German pathologist from Bonn, attempted to convince American physicians that "interstitial plasma cell pneumonia" was, in truth, not a virus infection but a *parasitic* infection. Hamperl's report was followed by a confirmatory paper by D. Carleton Gajdusek, published in 1957 in *Pediatrics* and entitled "*Pneumocystis carinii* — Etiologic agent of interstitial plasma cell pneumonia of premature and young infants."

Gajdusek had seen many cases of infantile Pneumocystis

pneumonia in hospitals in southern Germany, Switzerland, and Yugoslavia, during the postwar years between 1948 and 1952. Gajdusek also later uncovered cases of Pneumocystis pneumonia in children at the Royal Melbourne Hospital, in Melbourne, Australia.

Both Hamperl's and Gajdusek's reports alerted physicians to the frequent association of both *Pneumocystis carinii* and cytomegalovirus infection within the lungs of patients with "interstitial pneumonitis." This peculiar association of a parasite *and* a virus would continue to intrigue scientists studying the badly diseased lungs of AIDS patients dying with these two infectious agents.

Surprisingly, Hamperl was aware of only two adults with Pneumocystis pneumonia. Neither had evidence of cytomegalovirus infection. One patient was a 48 year-old man with leukemia. The other, a 21 year-old man whose cause of death was unknown. Hamperl seriously doubted that adults could get "pneumonitis" from cytomegalovirus alone. He believed that the Pneumocystis parasite was necessary to complete the infection.

To this day, many medical scientists recognize *Pneumocystis carinii* as a protozoan parasite, although there is no real proof of this. In order to study a microbe and to classify it with accuracy, it is necessary to grow it outside the body in "pure" culture.

While the epidemic of Pneumocystis pneumonia was raging in southern Europe in the 1950s, two Hungarian microbiologists were studying the parasite in Budapest. Anna Csillag, and L. Brandstein, succeeded in growing *Pneumocystis carinii* in artificial laboratory media, and claimed that the parasite was *not* a protozoan parasite but actually a yeast-like *fungus!*

Experimental laboratory rabbits and mice were forced to breathe aerosol sprays containing the parasites. In other experiments, the parasites were inserted into the windpipes of the animals. All the animals became ill and developed interstitial pneumonia. At the autopsies, the characteristic "spores" were observed in the animals' lungs. The two microbiologists were able to regrow the fungus from the lung tissue of the animals. Peculiarly, the animals which were treated with penicillin worsened and died sooner than animals who were untreated.

Other scientists have been unable to duplicate Csillag and Brandstein's experiments which indicated that Pneumocystis was a fungus-like microbe, rather than a protozoan parasite. The inability of microbiologists to grow *Pneumocystis carinii* in pure culture, has seriously limited animal research investigations. If animals could be experimentally infected with pure cultures of Pneumocystis parasites, much needed data might be obtained concerning the transmissibility of the disease, and new drugs and vaccines might be developed against the parasite.

Nevertheless, the animal experiments in Hungary, three decades ago, suggest that *Pneumocystis carinii* alone, (and without the addition of other infectious agents such as viruses), is capable of killing healthy animals. The treatment of Pneumocystis with certain antibiotics could worsen the experimental infection. Finally, the Hungarians pointed out that interstitial pneumonitis might be acquired from air-borne transmission of the parasite. This mode of transmission is quite different from all other protozoan parasitic diseases such as malaria, toxoplasmosis, amebiasis, giardiasis, and trypanosomiasis, which are *not* acquired by inhalation of the parasite (or by sexual intercourse).

Cases of "plasma cell interstitial pneumonia" in children, due to *Pneumocystis carinii*, were rarely reported in North America during the 1950s and 1960s. Occasional outbreaks occurred in premature and young infants. George Berdnikoff, a pathologist from Montreal, found fourteen cases in Canadian infants. He studied lung biopsy material from 3186 people, and found two cases of Pneumocystis pneumonia, dating back to 1930! Bernikoff claimed, in his 1959 report, that "the disease is much more common in this country, (Canada), than has been thought, and we have only to open our eyes to see it."

Particularly tragic and unusual examples of Pneumocystis lung infections were discovered in a family of three, from Washington state, and were reported by James Watanabe, *et al*, in 1965, in *The Journal of the American Medical Association*. A seven year-old girl became ill, in June 1964, with fever and breathing difficulties. The child's illness was treated as a "cold," but she worsened, with a persistent cough. In July, a chest X-ray showed "diffuse densities" in the lungs. The child was given antibiotics, and she slowly recovered, over the next few months.

In August, during the child's illness, her mother, age 22, also developed a cough, along with persistent fever. Despite penicillin, her cough worsened, and her breathing became more difficult. She was hospitalized on September 4, 1964. The chest X-ray showed "extensive infiltrates of the lungs." Despite additional antibiotics, she became increasingly cyanotic. Six days later, she died. The pathologist discovered *Pneumocystis carinii* in her lungs.

The story was to become more bizarre. In April 1964, two months before the child became ill, and five months before her mother's death, the child's father had been hospitalized with the "flu" and "atypical pneumonia." While the father was hospitalized, the doctors discovered he had acute leukemia. He was given a cortisone drug, and chemotherapy, for cancer. He did well on medication and returned home, and resumed working. However, at the end of August, he redeveloped a severe respiratory illness. He was hospitalized the day after his wife died. His chest X-ray showed similar "infiltrates," in the lungs. Nine days later, he was dead with Pneumocystis pneumonia. No virus was isolated from the lung tissue.

Currently, in the AIDS epidemic, *Pneumocystis carinii* is considered to be an opportunistic microbe, attacking people who are immunodepressed. But in 1965, Watanabe *et al* wrote that *"Pneumocystis carinii* is not necessarily opportunistic. *Pneumocystis carinii* pneumonia involved a young father and mother and presumably their daughter. The father had acute leukemia in remission, but the mother and daughter had been in prior good health. The father and mother died of their illness; the child survived. *Pneumocystis carinii* can occur in heretofore healthy adults and early diagnosis is important."

During the 1970s, it was becoming clear that children with cancer, especially those hospitalized and treated with chemotherapy, were prone to develop Pneumocystis pneumonia.

In 1973, a report from St. Jude Children's Research Hospital in Memphis, Tennessee, indicated that fifty one cases of Pneumocystis pneumonia had been diagnosed at the hospital. Forty eight cases had been discovered between 1968 and 1971. All these children had cancer. *Pneumocystis carinii* pneumonitis had occurred in over 4% of hospitalized children with cancer. The study concluded that Pneumocystis lung infections were possibly related to the prolonged survival of the cancer cases due to chemotherapy. "Accordingly, with the advances in cancer chemotherapy, prolonged survival, and the increase in 5 year cure rates, the high risk population will increase. *Opportunistic infections such as Pneumocystis carinii pneumonitis can be expected to be encountered more frequently.*" (Author's italics).

In 1975, another cluster of Pneumocystis lung infections, in cancer patients, occurred at the Memorial Sloan-Kettering Hospital, in New York City. This same hospital would later be reporting a substantial number of AIDS cases in homosexual men, apparently caused by a sexually transmitted virus.

Also in 1975, another outbreak of Pneumocystis pneumonia occurred in ten children, all with acute lymphoblastic leukemia, at the James Whitcomb Riley Hospital for Children, in Indianapolis, Indiana. Special serum blood testing of hospital personnel, and other epidemiologic data, indicated that the source and spread of the disease may have originated within the hospital environment.

In 1978, another provocative report from St. Jude

Children's Hospital, by Linda Pifer *et al*, indicated that Pneumocystis infection "is highly prevalent in *normal* children, with approximately 75% acquiring the infection by four years of age." The researchers had first grown the Pneumocystis organisms in the lungs of embryonated chickens. A purified "antigen" was made from the microbes. This antigen enabled the researchers to detect antibodies within the serum, of both healthy and sick children, who had been exposed to the Pneumocystis parasite.

The results of this immunologic blood testing indicated that "latent" infection (i.e. producing no symptoms) with *Pneumocystis carinii* is common in children. This latent lung infection also might explain why Pneumocystis organisms were occasionally found in the lungs of patients who showed no evidence of actual disease. The report suggested that immunosuppressive drugs and agents might "provoke or permit the activation of latent organisms, leading to replication and establishment of the disease process."

Pifer's group raised important questions about Pneumocystis infection. Does the microbe produce disease other than pneumonitis? How is the disease transmitted? Does Pneumocystis infection in older children and adults result from reactivation of an "old" latent infection, or is the lung infection acquired from "new" contact with the parasite? These questions would remain unanswered five years later in the AIDS crisis.

By the end of the 1970s, it was clear to scientists that *Pneumocystis carinii* pneumonia was a world-wide problem. Although epidemics of the disease were not recorded in Europe, after the mid-1950s, sporadic cases continued to be reported from Europe, Australia, New Zealand, Israel, Iran, Korea, Japan, Vietnam, and South America.

By 1980, a year before the AIDS epidemic was to explode in America, a short report, entitled "Pneumocystis pneumonia in hospitals: Outbreaks or improved recognition?", concluded that Pneumocystis is a frequent cause of pneumonia in immunosuppressed children, especially those with cancer. "All the outbreaks in the United States had occurred in the past 12 years, since the introduction of intensive chemo-therapy for leukemia and lymphoma. The increasing number of cases, after 1976, is probably due, in part, to the improvement in tumor therapy." It was not known how the disease was transmitted, but person-to-person transmission was a possibility. The development of new surgical biopsy techniques such as "percutaneous needle aspiration of the lung," were making it easier for doctors to secure lung tissue in order to diagnose Pneumocystis infection in ill patients with pneumonia.

The AIDS epidemic officially began in June 1981, when the CDC first reported cases of *Pneumocystis carinii* pneumonia in homosexual men hospitalized at the University of California Medical Center, at Los Angeles (UCLA). All the men had been studied by Michael Gottlieb, an allergist and immunologist, who was the first to suspect a possible epidemic of Pneumocystis pneumonia in gay men.

Gottlieb's original cases of interstitial pneumonia were described in great detail in *The New England Journal of Medicine*, (December 10, 1981). All four young men had been previously healthy, before acquiring Pneumocystis pneumonia. Three men had had fevers, for weeks, before the onset of the lung infection. White patches, characteristic of Candida yeast infection, were present in their mouths. Cytomegalovirus could be recovered from the men's secretions.

A detailed and research-oriented study of the men's white blood cells yielded remarkable and unique findings. The white blood counts were low. But peculiarly, the "helper T cell" level of the blood was dangerously depressed. T cells are special white blood cell lymphocytes needed to ward off infections and dangerous microbes, such as bacteria, viruses, and parasites.

What was causing this severe immunodeficiency? Gottlieb, and his colleagues at UCLA, attempted to explain the cause of the as-yet-unnamed epidemic in this way. Infection with cytomegalovirus was widespread within the male homosexual community. The virus could be sexually transmitted from person-to-person. All Gottlieb's patients had evidence of infection with this virus. Experience with laboratory animals experimentally-infected with cytomegalovirus had already shown that the virus could produce severe immunodepression.

Gottlieb's group concluded: "We acknowledge the possibility that cytomegalovirus infection was a result, rather than the cause, of the T cell defect, and that some other exposure to an undetected microorganism, drug, or toxin made these patients susceptible to infection with opportunistic organisms, including cytomegalovirus. However, at this time, cytomegalovirus is highly suspect, in view of its prevalence among male homosexuals, and its previously documented potential for immunosuppression."

One year later, Gottlieb was to further refine his views by suggesting that AIDS could result from not one, *but two* microbial infections. The first "initial" infection, probably a virus, causes depression of T cell immunity. This "initial suppression opens the door for a second infection or viral-associated malignancy." The second infection may be viral, protozoal, fungal, or mycobacterial; the nature of this secondary infection then determines whether the patient develops Kaposi's sarcoma, *Pneumocystis carinii* pneumonia, or any of several other opportunistic infections.

Following Gottlieb's article in the same issue of *The New England Journal of Medicine*, Henry Masur, *et al*, reported eleven additional cases of "community acquired" Pneumocystis pneumonia in adult men, from New York City. Six were homosexual; seven were drug abusers. Eight men had already died. Only two of five homosexuals had blood serologic evidence of cytomegalovirus infection.

Stephen Follansbee, *et al* (1982), reported five more cases of Pneumocystis pneumonia in homosexual men in San Francisco. Four had already died. All showed evidence of cytomegalovirus infection. Dorothy McCauley, *et al* (1982), recorded thirty gay men from New York City, with Pneumocystis pneumonia. Seventeen men also had Kaposi's sarcoma. Microscopic evidence of cytomegalovirus lung infection could be found in only one patient.

Gordon Gamsu, *et al* (1982), reported twelve homosexual men with Pneumocystis pneumonia, from San Francisco. All showed evidence of past or present infection with cytomegalovirus. The physicians stressed the "ground glass" appearance of the lungs in the chest X-ray pictures, similar to the glassy appearance of the lungs of infants who died decades earlier, in Europe, with epidemic interstitial pneumonia.

The statistics were piling up at the CDC. The implications for gay men were frightening.

In September 1981, the CDC had recorded 49 cases of Pneumocystis pneumonia, and 11 cases of *both* Pneumocystis and Kaposi's sarcoma. All were men. Ninety four percent were homosexual, or bisexual. Most resided in New York City, Los Angeles, or San Francisco. By March 1982, 135 cases of Pneumocystis had been recorded. Twenty eight more men had Pneumocystis and cancer. By July 1983, the total number of AIDS cases was over 1800. Most of the fatal AIDS cases were dying of *Pneumocystis carinii* pneumonia. By December 1985, the total AIDS cases was over 15,000!

The history of parasitic lung infection with *Pneumocystis carinii* revealed a few clear facts. Most human beings are exposed to the parasite. Until the 1980s, most people who developed Pneumocystis lung infection were either newborns and infants, or children and adults with cancer. Epidemics of Pneumocystis pneumonia had already occurred in children's wards in Europe, and in "mini-epidemics" in children's cancer wards in hospitals in America.

The explosion of *both* Pneumocystis pneumonia and immunosuppression in gay men was unprecedented. Certainly, there was no clear evidence that *Pneumocystis carinii* infection could be sexually transmitted. Previous reports had indicated that Pneumocystis could attack healthy, normal people, but this was rare. What was causing the immunosuppression leading to severe infection in homosexual men? Most epidemiologists and medical researchers, searching for the cause of AIDS, were directing their attention to the cytomegalovirus.

References

Follansbee SE, Busch DF, Wofsy CB, *et al: An outbreak of Pneumocystis carinii pneumonia in homosexual men. Ann Intern Med 96: 705-712, 1982.*

CDC: *Pneumocystis pneumonia — Los Angeles. MMWR 30:250, 1981.*

Chagas C: *Nova tripanozomiaza humana. Estudios sobre a morfolojia e o coclo evulotivo do Schizotrypanum cruzi n. gen., n. sp., ajente etiologio de nova entidade morbida de homen. Mem Inst Oswaldo Cruz 3: 219, 1909.*

Carini A: *Formas de eschizogonia do Trypanozoma Lewisi. Comm soc Med Sao Paulo, p204, August 16, 1910.*

Delanoe P, and Delanoe M: *Sur les rapports des kystes de Carini chez les cobayes de la region de paris: absence de kystes chez d'autres animaux lapin, grenouille, 3 anguilles. Bull Soc Path Exot 7: 271, 1912.*

van der Meer G, and Brug SL: *Infection a Pneumocystis chez l'homme et chez les animaux. Ann Soc Belg Med Trop 22: 301, 1942.*

Gajdusek D: *Pneumocystis carinii - etiologic agent of interstitial plasma cell pneumonia of premature and young infants. Pediatrics 19: 543-565, 1957.*

Vanek J: *Atypical interstitial pneumonia of infants produced by Pneumocystis carinii. Casop Lek Cesk 90: 1121, 1951.*

Vanek J: *Parasitic pneumonia due to Pneumocystis carinii in a 60 year-old woman. Casop Lek Cesk 91: 1260, 1951.*

Deamer WC, and Zollinger HU: *Interstitial "plasma cell" pneumonia of premature and young infants. Pediatrics 12: 11-22, 1953.*

Lunseth JH, Kirmse TW, Prezyna AP, *et al: Interstitial plasma cell pneumonia. Pediatrics 46: 137-145, 1955.*

Hamperl H: *Pneumocystis infection and cytomegaly of the lungs in the newborn and adult. Amer J Pathol 32: 1-13, 1956.*

Csillag A, and Brandstein L: *The role of Blastomyces species in the genesis of interstitial pneumonia of the premature infant. Acta Microb Hung 1: 525-529, 1954.*

Csillag A, and Brandstein L: *The role of blastomyces in the aetiology of interstitial pneumonia of the premature infant. Acta Microb Hung 2: 179-190, 1954.*

Berdnikoff G: *Fourteen cases of Pneumocystis carinii pneumonia. Canad Med J 80: 1-5, 1959.*

Watanabe JM, Clinchinian H, Weitz, C, *et al: Pneumocystis carinii pneumonia in a family. JAMA 193: 685-686, 1965.*

Hughes WT, Price RA, Kim HK, *et al: Pneumocystis carinii pneumonia in children with malignancies. J Pediatrics 82: 404-415, 1973.*

Ruebush TK, Weinstein RA, Bachner RL, *et al: An outbreak of Pneumocystis pneumonia in children with acute lymphocytic leukemia. Amer J Dis Child 132: 143-148, 1978.*

Pifer LL, Hughes WT, Stagno S, *et al: Pneumocystis carinii infection: Evidence for high prevalence in normal and immunosuppressed children. Pediatrics 61: 35-41, 1978.*

Gottlieb MS, Schroff R, Schanker HM, *et al: Pneumocystis carinii pneumonia and mucosal candidiasis in previously healthy homosexual men. N Engl J Med 305: 1431-1438, 1981.*

Gottlieb MS: *Ongoing AIDS epidemic could be product of dual pathogen infection. Skin and Allergy News 14: January, 1983.*

Masur H, Michelis MA, Greene JB, *et al: An outbreak of community acquired Pneumocystis carinii pneumonia. N Engl J Med 305: 1431-1438, 1981.*

McCauley DI, Naidich DP, Leitman BS, *et al: Radiographic patterns of opportunistic lung infections and Kaposi's sarcoma in homosexual men. Amer J Roentgenology 139: 653-656, 1982.*

Gamsu G, Hecht ST, Birnberg FA, *et al: Pneumocystis carinii pneumonia in homosexual men. Amer J Roentgenology 139: 647-651, 1982.*

DeWys WD, Curran J, Henle W, *et al: Workshop on Kaposi's sarcoma: Meeting report. Cancer Treat Rep 66: 1387-1390, 1982.*

Levine AS: *The epidemic of acquired immune dysfunction in homosexual men and its sequelae — opportunistic infections, Kaposi's sarcoma, and other malignancies: An update and interpretation. Cancer Treat Rep 66: 1391-1395, 1982.*

6 AIDS in Africa and Europe

"Anybody expecting hopeful news from the AIDS Conference held in New York, November 14-17, 1983, was in for a jolt. But scientists from Belgium and France unloaded some observations (not new) that prompted newspaper stories on both coasts suggesting that AIDS began in Africa. A group of researchers from the CDC had joined several Western Europeans earlier in 1983 on an exploratory mission to Kinshasa, the capital of Zaire. In the city's only hospital, they came upon about 50 cases of AIDS almost immediately. They found more in Rwanda, Chad, and Burundi. Most of the African cases seem to have no connection to the standard 'risk group' identification. Total mystery."
— Nathan Fain's "Health" column. The Advocate, January 10, 1984.

Although the AIDS epidemic officially began in America in June 1981, there are case reports in the medical literature, which suggest that some people in other parts of the world had acquired AIDS-like illnesses before that time.

The following reports are not intended to suggest that AIDS started in Africa or Europe. On the contrary, it is far more likely that AIDS has been, and will prove to be, a world-wide disease. The *recognition* of AIDS is undoubtedly a "new" phenomenon. However, the recorded cases cited in this chapter could serve as examples to show that *all* people, regardless of race or sexual preference, may be at risk for AIDS.

Kinshasa, Zaire (Africa), 1977

She was despondent about the poor health of her sixth child, her beautiful three month-old baby girl. She had three healthy children from her first marriage, but the next three children, which she bore from her second husband, had brought her unbearable sorrow and tragedy. Her fourth and fifth child had died in infancy; one of pneumonia, the other of a blood infection. Before their fatal illnesses, she had seen white patches in their mouths. To her dismay, her new daughter was born with similar white patches.

She knew what she must do. She was 36 years old. She had a good job as a secretary with the best airline company in Zaire, and her family was better off than most black families in Kinshasa. She would take her child to Belgium for treatment.

In August 1977, Belgian doctors at St. Raphael University Hospital, in Leuven, diagnosed the infant as immunodepressed. She was greatly relieved when the doctors said the baby would be all right with treatment.

But she was also mentally and physically exhausted, and she was experiencing fevers and constant headaches. The Belgian doctors discovered she was anemic. White patches appeared in her mouth. Her illness worsened. She was admitted to the University hospital in September, with fever, diarrhea, joint pains, swollen glands, and a lung infection. Over the next four months, her body was racked with repeated viral, bacterial, and yeast infections. Her liver and lymph glands became infected with a rare fungus called *Cryptococcus neoformans*. By January, she begged to go home to her family in Zaire. She died a month later in Kinshasa, in February 1978.

This case was reported in April 1983. The Belgian physicians wrote: "Three independent groups in Paris and Brussels have recently reported on severe opportunistic infections in previously healthy Africans, immigrants or not, without history of drug abuse, transfusions, or homosexuality. In all three reports these were patients from Zaire and it was suggested that Central Africa might be an endemic zone for the supposed infectious agent(s) of AIDS. Over the past two years at least a dozen Zairian patients have been admitted to hospitals in Belgium with clinical features suggestive of AIDS. Cryptococcosis was the most prominent opportunistic infection. Since only the better off families of Zaire can afford medical care in Europe these patients may be just the tip of the epidemiological iceberg. For about two years there has been a sharp increase in cryptococcosis in the major hospitals of Kinshasa. In the Mama Yemo General Hospital fifteen patients with cryptococcal meningitis were diagnosed over a period of 18 months, an incidence not previously recorded in Kinshasa."

Another case of a married, 23 year-old black Zairian woman with AIDS, was reported in March 1983. One week after arrival in Belgium in June 1981, she became acutely ill with fever, weakness, and swollen glands. A lymph node biopsy showed tuberculosis. The woman was treated for tuberculosis and recovered. In January 1982, she entered a Paris hospital with a lung infection. Pneumocystis parasites were found. She responded well to treatment, but was readmitted to the hospital two months later with a blood infection. She died four days later. At the autopsy, the pathologist found fungal microbes, (*Cryptococcus neoformans*), which had infected her liver, spleen, and lymph glands. Virus cultures were negative. The French doctors reporting the case emphasized that not all AIDS patients were homosexuals or drug abusers.

Zaire, Africa, 1976

A 42 year-old Danish surgeon came to work among the poor in a primitive rural hospital in northern Zaire in 1972. She stayed 5 years. During this time she was plagued with recurring attacks of diarrhea. In 1976, the doctor began to lose weight and to tire easily. Her lymph glands enlarged. While on vacation in South Africa in July 1977, she developed a severe respiratory illness. She was flown back to Denmark, and entered a Copenhagen hospital.

A lung biopsy showed *Pneumocystis carinii* parasites. She was given prednisone (cortisone), and oxygen. She improved enough to leave the hospital, but was readmitted with pneumonia in November 1977. White patches of a Candida yeast infection appeared in her mouth. A staphylococcal bacterial infection was found in her blood stream. Her breathing steadily worsened, and she died one month later, at age forty seven.

This case was reported by I. C. Bygbjerg, in April 1983, who wrote that "she could recall coming across at least one case of Kaposi's sarcoma while working in northern Zaire, and while working as a surgeon under primitive conditions she must have been heavily exposed to blood and excretions of African patients. She had not been to the USA or to Haiti, and did not abuse drugs."

Bygbjerg, who had worked in Zaire in 1976, remarked that "little attention has been paid to the hyperendemic focus of Kaposi's sarcoma in central Africa. Cases of AIDS without Kaposi's sarcoma stand little chance of being detected locally because immunological laboratories are not available."

Cologne, Germany, 1976

He was 49 years old in December 1976. His health had always been perfect, but lately, for some unknown reason, he felt constantly tired and weak. He assumed the bluish spots on his thigh were age spots, another sign that he was getting older. His doctor told him he was mildly anemic, and prescribed iron tablets. By summer, the anemia worsened, and a bone marrow test was ordered. The report indicated that the marrow was not producing enough red blood cells. A skin biopsy of a blue lesion showed Kaposi's sarcoma. To make matters worse, warts were developing around his anus.

In March 1978, he almost died of meningitis. By summer, his lymph glands had greatly enlarged. His bone marrow was producing less and less blood. He died in January 1979.

Doctors at the University at Cologne had previously reported this case in a German medical journal, but in 1983 they reported it again in *The Lancet*. They wrote: "We did not mention that this patient was homosexual because it did not seem relevant at the time. Because this case may have important implications for our thinking about the onset and spread of the AIDS epidemic, we think it worthwhile drawing attention to this case. The patient's Kaposi's sarcoma and homosexuality may have been fortuitous and unrelated to the current epidemic of AIDS, or his Kaposi's sarcoma may have been a consequence of AIDS, a hypothesis supported by the non-bacterial meningitis and perianal condylomata (warts). AIDS - related Kaposi's sarcoma may have existed in Europe and elsewhere before 1979, a view that corresponds with the lack of contact with Americans in some European cases of AIDS. The AIDS epidemic in the United States may indicate, not the appearance of a new infective agent, but merely the introduction of an old pathogen into a group of people whose promiscuous lifestyle would ensure rapid spread of infection or who had additional co-factors which increased the severity of infection."

Paris, France, 1981

The first French case of AIDS in a young homosexual man was reported in 1981. By December 1982, another Paris report confirmed twenty nine more AIDS cases, of which five cases were women; five were Haitian and Zairian. Many, but not all, of the French patients had traveled to the United States, Africa, or Haiti. The reporters suggested the "Equitorial Africa is an endemic zone for the supposed infectious agent(s) of the illness. Nine cases of what is now called AIDS were seen before June 1981, the date of the first report of the syndrome in the USA. This suggests that the illness and the supposed infectious agent(s) are not new in France. Only its recent epidemiologic features, in the USA and by the same token in France, are new."

Arkadi Rylwin, *et al*, reported the case of a fifty year-old black woman, ill for three months with fever, chills, extreme fatigue, and weight loss. The woman's liver, spleen, and lymph glands were enlarged, and she had abnormal immunologic tests. It was thought she had lymph gland cancer (lymphoma), and a possible heart infection. She was hospitalized, and treated with antibiotics and chemotherapy. The fever continued daily. She went into heart failure, and died one month later. At the autopsy, the pathologist found tumors of Kaposi's sarcoma in her stomach, intestines, and adrenal glands.

Amazingly, two other patients at the same hospital had shown the same illness. Both were Jewish men in their seventies. These two white men, and the black woman, were all patients who had fever, weight loss, immunologic abnormalities, and enlargement of the liver, spleen, and lymph nodes. All died of Kaposi's sarcoma within seven months of their illnesses. *Strangely, none had skin tumors of Kaposi's sarcoma!* The reporting doctors noted the similarity of these three rapidly fatal cases to previously described cases of African Kaposi's sarcoma, occurring in black children and young adults, in which external tumors were seldom present.

Today, the two Jewish men could never qualify as having AIDS. They were simply too old. According to current CDC criteria for the diagnosis of AIDS, cases of Kaposi's sarcoma must be under the age of sixty. The fifty year-old black woman would certainly have AIDS if diagnosed today.

But these three rare cases, strangely reminiscent of AIDS-like illnesses, and African Kaposi's sarcoma, were diagnosed in a Miami, Florida, hospital in the early 1960s. The report was certainly evidence that the African type of Kaposi's sarcoma existed, in America, two decades before the "Gay" AIDS epidemic officially started in 1981.

In June 1983, the first suspected cases of AIDS in Australia were reported in *The Medical Journal of Australia*. The cover of the journal showed a human skull, and an X-ray picture of the diseased lungs of a twenty seven year-old, gay American man. The man had lived in Sydney for only a few weeks before developing a life-threatening respiratory illness.

Two captions also appeared on the journal cover. One referred to AIDS as "the black plague of the eighties..."; the other caption read, "Perhaps we've needed a situation like this to show us what we have known all along — DEPRAVITY KILLS!"

Fortunately, this young, immunodepressed man rapidly recovered from the acute lung disease with medication for "pneumocystis" pneumonia. However, it is unlikely that the CDC in America would accept this case as a *proven* AIDS patient because Australian doctors were unable to find pneumocystis parasites in the biopsy of lung tissue.

Nevertheless, Ronald Perry, and the other reporting physicians concluded that "we believe this patient represents the first Australian case of a new disease which has become known as AIDS." They recommended that "any male homosexuals visiting the United States of America should be strongly advised to refrain from sexual activity." Other reports, by Angus Dalgleish, *et al*, and Coleman Smith, *et al*, in this same issue, attested to four more cases of immunodepressed Australian gay men with unproven, but suspected "AIDS-like conditions," consisting of fever, weight loss, fatigue, and swollen glands.

By the summer of 1983, the CDC had accepted one case of AIDS from Japan, as well as one case from Argentina, and Brazil. It is now apparent that the 1981 epidemic of AIDS is a world-wide health problem. Scientists are still puzzled as to where in the world the epidemic initially began.

In his letter appearing in *The New England Journal of Medicine*, (September 15, 1983), Fritz Cineas, the Haitian ambassador to the United States, was obviously angry that Haiti had been selected "as a scapegoat for a mysterious ailment that has, sadly, descended upon the American homosexual community." Cineas claimed that "the Republic of Haiti has suffered a severe injustice over the past year in the American press. The time is well overdue for the record to be set straight regarding AIDS and the Haitian connection. I am sure a responsible institution like yours will uphold your admirable American tradition of unveiling the truth."

Clearly, Cineas was objecting to the so-called "Haitian connection" to AIDS, which we will next examine.

References

Vandepitte J, Verwilghen R, Zachee P: *AIDS and cryptococcosis (Zaire, 1977). Lancet 1:924-925, 1983.*

Offenstadt G, Pinta P, Hericord P, *et al: Multiple opportunistic infection due to AIDS in a previously healthy black woman from Zaire. New Engl J Med 308: 775, 1983.*

Clumeck N, Mascart-Lemone F, de Maubeuge J, *et al: Acquired immune deficiency syndrome in black Africans. Lancet 1:642, 1983.*

Bygbjerg IC: *AIDS in a Danish surgeon (Zaire, 1976). Lancet 1:925, 1983.*

Sterry W, Marmor M, Konrads A, *et al: Kaposi's sarcoma, aplastic pancytopenia, and multiple infections in a homosexual (Cologne, 1976). Lancet 1: 924-925, 1983.*

Brunet JB, Bouvet E, Chaperon J, *et al: Acquired immunodeficiency syndrome in France. Lancet 1:700-701, 1983.*

Rywlin AM, Recher L, Hoffman EP: *Lymphoma-like presentation of Kaposi's sarcoma. Arch Dermatol 93: 554-561, 1966.*

Perry R, Marks R, Berger J, *et al: Acquired immune deficiency syndrome. Med J Austral 1:554-557, 1983.*

Dalgleish AG, Prentice KL, Gatenby PA, *et al: Acquired immune deficiency syndrome. A prodromal form. Med J Austral 1:558-560, 1983.*

Smith CI, Motum PI, Wall RS: *Prodromal acquired immune deficiency syndrome in Australian homosexual men. Med J Austral 1:561-563, 1983.*

Cineas FN: *Haitian ambassador deplores AIDS connection. New Engl J Med 309: 668-669, 1983.*

7 AIDS: The Haitian Connection

It is unlikely scientists will ever determine the country or region where the AIDS epidemic originated. At the end of the fifteenth century when epidemics of syphilis first erupted in Europe, Italians blamed the French for starting the epidemic. Needless to say, the French blamed the Italians, and so on.

The Spaniards were convinced the new and sometimes fatal disease had been brought to Europe by Columbus and his sailors, on their return from the island of Hispanola (now Haiti), in the West Indies. The source of the syphilis epidemic was assumed to be the New World, and the spreaders were the "red" Indians of Hispanola. Five centuries later, some epidemiologists were suspecting the AIDS epidemic in America originated among the now black population of Haiti.

Haitians in America are currently one of the groups at risk for AIDS. Poor, uneducated, and recently arrived Haitian immigrants with AIDS, not only have to face the gloomy prognosis of their illness, but must also cope with a language they often do not understand, as well as the added social pressures which always affect persons afflicted with an epidemic and contagious disease.

Some Haitian doctors have claimed AIDS did not exist in Haiti before 1981. Haitian immigrants with AIDS have repeatedly denied homosexuality and drug abuse. However, Nathan Fain in his "Health" column in *The Advocate*, (August 4, 1983), indicated there might be some inaccuracies about Haitians. By June (1983), confirmed reports, from both Haitian and non-Haitian physicians, were suggesting some Haitian men with AIDS "had engaged in homosexual sex, often for hire." Although homosexuality is taboo in Haitian society, Jean Claude Des Granges of the Haitian Medical Association had discovered a suburb in Port-au-Prince "that resembles New York's Times Square in its open licentiousness" and where "prostitution of both sexes was practiced."

By the summer of 1983, the New York City Health Department (but not the CDC) dropped Haitians from the "high risk" group for AIDS. The Department was convinced that many Haitians with AIDS were homosexual or intravenous drug abusers. Nevertheless, many people still held Haiti and the Haitians responsible for the "spread" of AIDS to America.

Georges was twenty seven years-old when he left France in 1978 to work in Haiti as a geologist. He was there for eight months when he was almost killed in an auto accident. His left arm was amputated. Eight units of Haitian blood were transfused into his body. When he recovered, he returned to France.

Three years later, diarrhea, abdominal pain, and fever began. By March 1982, Georges had lost 22 pounds, and was told he had AIDS. But that was *impossible*. He wasn't gay. He had a healthy wife and child, never took drugs, and had always been well except for the horrible accident in Haiti.

There were no swollen glands, and no sign of Kaposi's sarcoma skin tumors. But he was profoundly immunodeficient. The bowel tests showed intestinal infection with "protozoan parasites" called *Cryptosporidium*. Despite medication, his condition worsened.

Two months later, Georges experienced the first of many

blood infections with a bacterium called *Salmonella typhimurium*. By autumn 1983, he had a stroke, and a brain abscess caused by another parasite, (*Toxoplasma gondii*). He developed high fevers, drifted into a coma, and died. The family refused an autopsy examination.

Georges' case met the CDC criteria for AIDS. He had no previous immunologic defect, and no known drug history. He was severely immunodepressed and had multiple opportunistic infections. The French doctors pointed out that "most individuals with AIDS are homosexual or bisexual young men," and "Haiti is a favorite vacation spot for many US homosexual men." But they also suspected a transmissible agent might have been acquired from Haitian blood. If so, the incubation period for AIDS could be as long as four years.

———————

The so-called "Haitian connection" cannot be understood without some knowledge of Haiti. Haiti is the poorest country in the western hemisphere. The black population is largely descended from slaves, brought from West Africa to Haiti, as early as the sixteenth century. The current average annual income is $300. According to Michele Barry, *et al* (1980), this poverty contributes significantly to Haiti's endemic diseases such as tuberculosis, typhoid fever, bacterial and protozoal dysenteries, malaria, and widespread malnutrition. Until the 1950s, tuberculosis was the major cause of death in Haitian hospitals. As late as 1950, there were only twenty six physicians for the total population of 2.5 million people. This shortage of physicians was compounded by the fact that over 70% of Haitian doctors emigrated. A 1969 law forbade further emigration without authorization.

In 1954, almost 90% of the Haitian population were given "long-acting penicillin therapy" for the treatment and eradication of yaws, an infectious disease caused by bacteria similar, but not identical, to the bacteria that cause syphilis.

By the summer of 1982, one year after the "Gay" epidemic began, the first 34 cases of AIDS in Haitian immigrants were reported by the CDC. Haitians were found to comprise 6% of all AIDS cases, in America. All the Haitian patients denied homosexuality and drug abuse. Details of some of these patients were published in 1983.

Jeffrey Vieira, *et al* (1983), reported ten previously healthy heterosexual Haitian men with AIDS from the New York City area. Six had tuberculosis, due to *Mycobacterium tuberculosis*. Other opportunistic infections included the parasite *Toxoplasmosis gondii* (4 cases); *Pneumocystis carinii* (4 cases); the yeast *Candida albicans* (3 cases); and a fungus *Cryptococcus neoformans* (1 case). All were immunodepressed. Six men died.

Twenty Haitians (17 men; 3 women) with AIDS were also reported from the Miami, Florida, area by Arthur Pitchenik, *et al* (1983). All had one or more opportunistic infections. One patient had Kaposi's sarcoma. Seven patients had tuberculosis, which developed two to fifteen months before AIDS. The tuberculosis was thought to be "secondary to T cell immunodeficiency."

The high incidence of tuberculosis in Haitian immigrants with AIDS should not be surprising, due to the high incidence of TB in Haiti. Pitchenik, in a later interview, stressed that not all Haitians with AIDS were recent immigrants. Some had been in the Miami area for as long as 7 years. He also stated "my opinion is not that tuberculosis predisposes to AIDS but that among Haitians it's often an early manifestation of the immunodeficiency syndrome. We see disseminated tuberculosis among all groups, but much more among the Haitians."

The issue of mycobacterial and "atypical" mycobacterial infection in AIDS, as possible *causative* agents in AIDS, is vitally important. Although the mycobacterium that causes tuberculosis was discovered over a century ago, many scientists and physicians have not stressed that typical and atypical tuberculosis infection can *in itself cause immunosuppression*. In addition, some chemothera-peutic *drugs* in the treatment of TB *can also cause immunosuppression*.

Guy Youmans, in his book "Tuberculosis" (1979), empha-sizes that tuberculosis bacteria can remain "dormant within tissues of human beings for many months, for years, or even a lifetime." Immunosuppression in tuberculosis is common, and can have a "suppressive effect on cellular immunity and upon the capacity of a person to mount an adequate defense to the invading microorganisms."

According to Sheldon Landesman, of the New York Downstate Medical Center in Brooklyn, about 20% of Hai-tians in America who have tuberculosis later develop AIDS. The Haitian population in America is estimated to be about 500,000. As many as 400,000 are thought to be living in the Brooklyn and Queens boroughs of New York City. Newark, (New Jersey), and Miami have large Haitian populations. Twenty two cases of AIDS in Haitians have been diagnosed in Brooklyn; twenty five cases in Miami.

The relationship between epidemiologic factors in AIDS, such as immunosuppression, mycobacterial infection and tuberculosis, Kaposi's sarcoma, opportunistic infection, het-erosexuality, promiscuity, contagion, and international tra-vel, can be vividly brought to life in the following Paris report by Tony Dournon, *et al* (1983), entitled "AIDS in a Haitian couple in Paris."

A thirty one year-old Haitian woman had lived in Paris since August 1979. She became ill with weakness, fever, and fatigue in February 1981. In August, she was hospital-ized due to immunodepression. Her condition deteriorated with a stroke, and a brain abscess. She died in February 1982. At the autopsy, it was discovered that a protozoan par-asite, (*Toxoplasmosis gondii*), had infected the brain.

Her Haitian husband, age thirty eight, had never been to America. He arrived in Paris, in October 1981, during his wife's illness. A year later, he was admitted to the *same* hospital with immunodepression, diarrhea, and a bacterial infection of the blood, caused by *Aeromonas hydrophilia*. Doctors also found tuberculosis of the lung. The bacterium causing the TB, (*Mycobacterium tuberculosis*), was grown from his sputum, liver, and bone marrow. Despite treatment, he died four months later with "overwhelming infection with culture-proven cytomegalovirus." At the autopsy, Kaposi's sarcoma was found in his lymph nodes.

The wife also had had tuberculosis in 1974. Two years before her death in Paris, she had lived for nine months in Newark, New Jersey. During this time away from Paris, she had a sexual relationship with a Haitian man, who later also developed AIDS. Although she previously had tuberculosis, her TB skin test was negative when tested in Paris. Her husband's skin test was also negative, even though he had "active" tuberculosis at the time.

Doctors rely heavily on "positive" TB skin tests to diagnose active or inactive tuberculosis. It used to be thought *all* persons with tuberculosis would have positive skin tests. However, some people with tuberculosis simply do not react to skin testing. The reason for this is that tuberculosis is an immunosuppression disease. In AIDS patients, skin tests for tuberculosis are almost always negative. But, despite a "negative" TB skin test, some of these patients may actually be dying of tuberculosis!

According to Youmans, the erroneous interpretation of TB skin test results "has led to some tragic errors in diagnosis in which persons with negative tuberculin tests, but with widespread tuberculosis, have not received chemotherapy because in view of a negative tuberculin test, it was thought that the disease must have another etiology." Despite the fact that tuberculosis may result in immunosuppression, the French doctors reported that the Haitian couple had "no previous illnesses associated with immunodepression."

Although the ability of viruses to cause immunodepression in AIDS has been highly touted by research scientists, little attention has been paid to mycobacteria, and other bacteria, which can also cause serious immunosuppression in human beings.

Three years after the beginning of the AIDS epidemic, epidemiologists were still trying to determine if AIDS had started in America, or in Haiti. To complicate matters, a few cases of Kaposi's sarcoma had been discovered in Haiti. In an interview appearing in *Skin and Allergy News*, (October 1983), Ary Bordes, the Haitian Minister of Health, claimed "the reluctance of Haitians to admit that they are homosexual or drug abusers, is responsible for their erroneous placement on the list of high risk groups for AIDS." Bordes was also quoted as saying that there were *157 known cases of AIDS in Haiti, as of August 1983*!

By 1984, Haitians were bitterly resenting their inclusion in the "4 H" club, a new and derisive term bantered about in the scientific community and the media, to denote the homosexuals, heroin abusers, hemophilics, and Haitians who comprised most of the AIDS cases.

To make matters worse, some newborns were coming down with AIDS in the New York City area. Some of these infants had Haitian parents.

References

Adreani T, Le Charpentier Y, Brouet JC, *et al: Acquired immunodeficiency with intestinal cryptosporidiosis: Possible transmission by Haitian whole blood. Lancet 1: 1187-1191, 1983.*

Barry M, Stansfield SK, Bia FJ: *Haiti and the Hospital Albert Schweitzer. Ann Intern Med 98: 1018-1020, 1983.*

Leonidas JR, and Hyppolyte N: *Haiti and the acquired immunodeficiency syndrome. Ann Intern Med 98: 1020-1021. 1983.*

CDC: *Opportunistic infections and Kaposi's sarcoma among Haitians in the United States. MMWR 31: 353-354, 360-361, 1982.*

Vieira J, Frank E, Spira TJ, *et al: Acquired immune deficiency in Haitians. New Engl J Med 308: 125-129, 1983.*

Pitchenik AE, Fischl MA, Dickenson GM, *et al: Opportunistic infections and Kaposi's sarcoma among Haitians: Evidence of a new acquired immunodeficiency state. Ann Intern Med 98: 277-284, 1983.*

Pitchenik AE: *AIDS among Haitians may not be limited to recent immigrants: Tuberculosis may be a marker for the syndrome in this group. Sex Trans Bull 3:4, 1983.*

Youmans GP: *Tuberculosis. WB Saunders Company, Philadelphia, 1979, pp 318-325.*

Landesman SH: *Haitian immigrants with tuberculosis might be prone to development of AIDS. Skin Allergy News 14:8, 1983.*

Dournon E, Penalba C, Wolff M, *et al: AIDS in a Haitian couple in Paris. Lancet 1: 1040-1041, 1983.*

8 PAIDS in Children

"Until recently, AIDS seemed to be limited to adults, predominantly those with aberrant life-styles, or exposure to blood products. It seems, however, that the epidemiology of AIDS may now have taken an ominous new turn, with otherwise 'normal' infants and children as additional victims." Oleske J, *et al:* Immune deficiency syndrome in children. The Journal of the American Medical Association, May 6, 1983.

By 1984, "baby doctors" (pediatricians) were becoming more and more convinced an infectious agent was being passed on to children. The source of the infection was either adults who had AIDS, or adults who were at risk for AIDS. Approximately fifty infants and children were suspected of having the syndrome. Pediatricians were calling the "new" disease — the "pediatric acquired immune deficiency syndrome" (PAIDS).

It was inevitable that an illness resembling AIDS would be discovered in newborns and in infants whose fragile and immature "immune systems" place them at risk for the development of many infectious diseases. Furthermore, an infectious microbe, such as the suspected infectious agent of AIDS, would hardly be expected to respect or to recognize age limits. Although the CDC was reticent about accepting adult cases of AIDS over the age of 60, the Center was avidly collecting data on possible cases of childhood AIDS.

In the May 6, 1983 issue of *The Journal of the American Medical Association*, two reports first suggested that infants could acquire AIDS. James Oleske, *et al*, described eight infants from the Newark, New Jersey area, who were born into families having one or more adult members with known risk factors for AIDS, such as heterosexual and homosexual intravenous drug abusers, Haitians/Dominicans, and prostitutes. All infants had "unexplained immunodeficiencies, some of whom had opportunistic infections and fit the working definition of AIDS developed by the CDC."

For many years it has been known that newborns could be affected with "congenital" immune deficiency diseases. However, these eight children had an illness that was believed to be "related in some way to household exposure, and their residence in communities involved in the current epidemic of AIDS."

All the infants had "interstitial pneumonia." Three infants died with Pneumocystis pneumonia. In one case, this parasite was discovered at the autopsy. The pediatricians considered that the AIDS-like illness might be the result of neglect, malnutrition, and socioeconomic conditions. However, it was still believed the children's illnesses were better diagnosed as AIDS-like disease.

The researchers rejected a "congenital" disease for two reasons. First, a "congenital defect would be expected to remain static." Second, "it is difficult for us to conclude that we and others have simultaneously experienced a sudden upsurge in congenital immune defects or congenital viral infections of the usual type."

The second report, by Arye Rubenstein, *et al*, described seven children from New York City. All developed the "new syndrome of acquired immunodeficiency" before the age of six months. Two of the seven were ill at birth. The mothers of five children were either sexually promiscuous, or drug addicts, or both. Three mothers were immunodeficient, and one mother eventually died of AIDS. All the children had "interstitial pneumonia," enlarged lymph nodes, and enlarged livers.

Five of the children, and three mothers, had evidence of infection with the "Epstein-Barr" virus. The doctors speculated this virus might have produced the AIDS-like disease. The virus could have been transmitted "vertically" from the mothers to their newborns.

In the editorial, Anthony Fauci, of the National Institutes of Health, commented on these two reports. "The difficulty that one faces in making a diagnosis of AIDS in an infant is related to the fact that a number of congenital immune deficiencies, and viral infections that result in immune deficiencies can be seen in infants and children. Therefore, it becomes difficult to ascertain that the syndrome is indeed acquired. The finding of AIDS in infants and children, who are household contacts of patients with AIDS or persons with risks for AIDS, has enormous implications with regard to ultimate transmissibility of this syndrome." Fauci emphasized "Again, I must reiterate the fact that we must be cautious in our acceptance of these infant cases as being truly AIDS."

All fifteen children included in these two reports had "interstitial pneumonia," and other physical and immunologic abnormalities. None had Kaposi's sarcoma. The pediatricians were apparently convinced they were seeing a "new" disease. Although three children had parasitic Pneumocystis pneumonia, no mention was made of epidemic cases of "infantile interstitial pneumonia," which had proved fatal to thousands of European children. One wonders if those European infants would be diagnosed as AIDS cases if they could be studied today in American hospitals.

AIDS-like illness in children is a serious and sometimes fatal disease. These two quoted studies most strongly suggest the transmission of the "AIDS microbe" from pregnant mothers to their newborns. Oleske's study indicated a few children with so-called AIDS could have healthy, "normal" parents. If so, then it is further evidence that the "AIDS microbe" can be present within the blood stream of *both* "normal" and "infected" mothers. Although maternal promiscuity during pregnancy might be a factor in childhood AIDS, promiscuity is hardly a new phenomenon accounting for the development of a "new" disease. However, drug addiction during pregnancy can produce disastrous effects on the fetus.

The general health of a newborn infant depends greatly upon the health of its mother, as well as the absence of infectious agents which could be passed from the mother's blood to the developing fetus. It is well-known that much of the newborn's "natural" immunity against infection is derived from maternal protective "antibodies." But it is also conceivable that a mother with active or "silent" AIDS could pass the infectious and "transmissible agent" of AIDS to her unborn child.

Some pediatricians, like Oleske, were still stressing the "homosexual connection" to childhood AIDS. In an interview in the *American Medical News*, (December 16, 1983), Oleske was quoted as saying that one key to the AIDS epidemic "may be the promiscuous bisexual male who is on drugs and who occasionally goes to the bathhouses as a male prostitute. He then contracts AIDS and passes it on to his wife who passes it on to the children. Most of these children are probably infected when passing through a contaminated birth canal or through the placental blood. That's as intimate as you can get without having sex."

By 1984, the recognition of fifty possible AIDS cases in children intensified the efforts of blood banks to discourage homosexuals from donating blood. One case of childhood AIDS received widespread media attention, even before the case was officially reported by Arthur Amman, *et al*, in 1983. In this case, an infant from San Francisco who had received multiple blood transfusions for anemia at birth, later died of AIDS, at age 20 months. One of the original blood donors, a healthy gay man at the time of his blood donation, also later died of AIDS. This, and other reports, contributed greatly to the public fear of AIDS. Some parents were making special efforts to keep their children away from known or suspected homosexuals, Haitians, and other "high risk" groups of people.

Pediatricians are searching diligently for a "new virus" as the most likely infectious agent of PAIDS. But as we will learn, all human beings, including unborn children, harbor potentially infectious bacteria within the blood stream. These microbes, already discovered, have been implicated not only in AIDS, but also in many forms of cancer (the second leading cause of death in children), Kaposi's sarcoma, "autoimmune" diseases, and a variety of other human illnesses.

References

Oleske J, Minnefor A. Cooper R Jr, *et al: Immune deficiency in children. JAMA 249: 2345-2349, 1983.*

Rubinstein A, Sicklick M, Gupta A, *et al: Acquired immunodeficiency with reversed T4/T8 ratios in infants born to promiscuous and drug-addicted mothers. JAMA 249: 2350-2356, 1983.*

Fauci AS: *The acquired immune deficiency syndrome. The ever-broadening clinical spectrum. JAMA 249: 2375-2376, 1983.*

Breo DL: *MD treats "innocent victims" of AIDS. American Medical News, December 16, 1983.*

Amman AJ, Cowan MJ, Wara DW, *et al: Acquired immunodeficiency in an infant: Possible transmission by means of blood products. Lancet 1: 956-958, 1983.*

Amman AJ, Wara DW, and Cowan MJ: *Pediatric Acquired Immonodeficiency Syndrome. Presented at a "Symposium of Immunodeficiency Diseases," Los Angeles Hilton, Los Angeles, December 9, 1983.*

9 The Immune System in AIDS and Cancer

Until the end of the eighteenth century, smallpox was one of the most feared epidemic diseases. Those who did not die were often left horribly disfigured, with pock-marked faces and bodies. Strangely, milkmaids, who frequently were exposed to "cowpox" sores, often seemed to be unaffected, or "immune" to the devastating effects of smallpox during outbreaks of the disease.

An English physician, Edward Jenner, first began to "vaccinate" people in 1796 against smallpox, by inoculating their skin with material from "cowpox" pustules. At the time, scientists knew nothing about microbes, or the immune system. But Jenner's crude "vaccine" was successful in protecting or "immunizing" people against smallpox, a disease now known to be caused by a virus. Vaccination was the first form of "preventive medicine" against infectious disease. A century later, Pasteur's vaccines, and Koch's microbiologic discoveries, were to revolutionize medical thought about infectious and epidemic diseases.

The dream of some scientists in this century is to produce a vaccine against cancer. Until a few decades ago, the idea was considered ridiculous. All cancers were believed to be noninfectious, and the body's immune system was thought to play no role in the development or spread of cancer.

Doctors reasoned that if a cancer tumor could metastasize

to other areas of the body, then the immune system was obviously of no importance in limiting the spread of cancer within the body. The idea of an "immune response" in cancer, didn't make sense. Scientists further theorized that the cancer cells would not produce irritants ("antigens") which would provoke the immune system to make "antibodies." These antibodies might be injurious to the cancer cells.

By the 1950s, scientists finally realized that human cancer *did* arouse a "specific immune response." Furthermore, the immune system could be studied and strengthened in cancer.

What is the "immune system?" Obviously, the *whole* body and *all* its cells are designed to assure the survival of human beings on this planet. Nevertheless, the "immune system" is currently regarded as the body's main defense system against invading microbes. The immune system is composed of the blood cells, the spleen (which filters and stores blood), the bone marrow (which produces blood), and the lymphatic system consisting of lymph nodes and their connecting lymph channels.

Within the immune system are two types of "white" blood cells, the so-called "B" and "T cells." B cells make "antibodies" which are protein-like immune substances found in the blood stream. T cells live for years, and help protect the tissue cells from harmful microbes such as viruses, bacteria, fungi, and parasites. T cells are further subdivided into "helper" (inducer) cells, and "suppressor" (cytotoxic) T cells.

Until the mid-1970s, scientists had not perfected the technology to detect these cells. Diagnostic testing for T and B cells is now possible. The cost is about $100. Abnormal test results of T and B cells can be found not only in AIDS patients, but also in patients with viral diseases, such as infectious hepatitis, infectious mononucleosis, and other infections.

In itself, the T and B cell test is *not* diagnostic of AIDS, but may predict persons at risk for AIDS. Along with other clinical and diagnostic tests, the T and B cell test is helpful in making a diagnosis of AIDS.

In "normal" people, there are twice as many helper cells than suppressor cells, making a "normal ratio" of 2 to 1. In AIDS, both helper and suppressor T cells are *decreased* in number. However, the helper cells are much more severely reduced in number than the suppressor cells. As a result, there is a marked imbalance between the two different types of T cells. Often, in AIDS, the actual number of helper and suppressor T cells are about equal, making a ratio of 1 to 1, instead of the normal ratio of 2 to 1. In severe cases of AIDS the ratio is much lower.

Healthy gay men who are sexually active may have *abnormal* T cell ratios. Similarly, female prostitutes may also have abnormal immunologic tests, and may also be at risk for AIDS. Surprisingly, a few gay men with Kaposi's sarcoma, and other AIDS-related illnesses, have been found to be immunologically *normal*.

However, on the basis of immunologic testing, and the high rate of cytomegalovirus infection in promiscuous homosexual men, many scientists now consider gay men to be abnormal immunologically unless proven otherwise. These scientific findings in AIDS have been widely publicized. As a result, the general public now also perceives gay men as biologically "different" from "normal" (heterosexual) people.

Unfortunately, medical scientists have not stressed that many cancer patients, and patients with chronic infectious diseases, may also have severe immunological abnormalities during these illnesses. The immunologic abnormalities in these non-AIDS patients have never been correlated with sexual activity and sexual orientation.

Most doctors now believe cancer can result from immunologic disturbances. Immunologic deficiencies are obviously more pronounced in certain kinds of cancers, than in others. Hugh Barber, in "Immunobiology for the Clinician" (1977), has written, "There are many factors which contribute to immunosuppression. Among these are aging, the neoplastic (cancerous) process *per se*, anticancer drug therapy, neonatal thymectomy, and, to a lesser extent, antibiotics, anesthetics, analgesics, and hypnotics. In reality, it is difficult to separate the contributions of drugs and disease in bringing about immunosuppression."

Hodgkin's disease is a rare form of lymphoma cancer, with severe immunologic abnormalities. Patients with this cancer are subject to severe opportunistic infections with viruses, bacteria, mycobacteria, fungi, yeast, and parasitic infections, identical to those infections seen in some AIDS patients. Despite epidemiological evidence suggesting "clusters" of certain cases of Hodgkin's disease, scientists have never believed the disease is due to a "sexually transmitted agent."

The role of opportunistic infection in *all* forms of cancer is also well-known. Jean Klastersky (1982), states that "infection is very common in patients with cancer. In addition, it is often severe, leading to substantial morbidity and mortality."

According to current CDC criteria, cancer patients, (except possibly for those with lymphomas), cannot ever be considered as possible AIDS patients. Similarly, patients receiving immunosuppressive drugs are also excluded from AIDS. This effectively removes most cancer patients from AIDS because chemotherapy, (and radiation therapy), is required treatment for many forms of cancer, including lymphomas. The immunologic results of T and B cell testing, in all forms and stages of "different" cancers are not known.

Aside from the results of immunologic testing, there are striking similarities between some "regular" cancer patients and AIDS cases, (with and without cancer). Both cancer and AIDS patients are at risk for added disease with a wide variety of infectious microbes. Both often lose tremendous amounts of weight, become "toxic," and die, in an emaciated state.

Many forms of cancer are now thought to be caused by viruses. Scientists have never cautioned people against "catching" cancer from sex. But scientists are now cautioning homosexuals about sexually transmitted viruses which are thought to cause Kaposi's sarcoma and AIDS. Why would cancer-producing viruses be active in the milieu of homosexual sex, and not be active in heterosexual sex? Before we discuss that issue, we should consider the proposed role of viruses in human cancer.

References

Barber HRK: *Immunobiology for the Clinician. John Wiley & Sons, New York, 1977, p 205.*

Kung PC, Berger CL, Estabrook A, *et al: Monoclonal antibodies for clinical investigation of human T lymphocytes. Intl J Dermatol 22:67-74, 1983.*

Wallace JI, Downes J, Ott A, *et al: T cell ratios in New York City prostitutes. Lancet 1: 58-59, 1983.*

Klastersky J: *Treatment of severe infections in patients with cancer. Arch Intern Med 142: 1984-1987, 1982.*

Campbell J: *AIDS Symposium revisited in New York, March 17-20, 1983. The BAPHRON 5:5, Supplement, May 1983.*

10   Viruses, AIDS, and Cancer

Although the cause of both AIDS and cancer is unknown, most scientists now believe viruses are the most likely agents of these diseases. What are viruses and how are they involved in the epidemic of AIDS?

Viruses are tinier than the smallest bacteria, and cannot be seen with an ordinary microscope. However, as a result of infection with certain viruses, the diseased tissue cells may produce viral "inclusion bodies," which can be identified microscopically.

Viruses are considered to be *non-living* particles composed of protein, or glycoprotein. All viruses contain a "core" of either DNA (desoxyribonucleic acid) or RNA (ribonucleic acid), but never both. Viruses can only reproduce within living cells. The details of how this is accomplished are not fully understood.

With the development of the electron microscope in Germany in the early 1940s, tissue could be magnified up to 200,000 times. This enabled scientists to finally *see* viruses.

The idea of viruses was proposed at the end of the nineteenth century. It was then known that certain infectious diseases could be transmitted by "filtered" and bacteria-free diseased tissue. Until the middle of this century, many scientists thought viruses were simply smaller forms of bacteria. Effective vaccines had already been developed for the prevention of some viral diseases, even though viruses had never been seen or grown. Many diseases including small-pox, rabies, influenza, poliomyelitis, measles, mumps, chicken pox, and hepatitis, are viral diseases.

For the first half of the twentieth century, most scientists were convinced that *all* forms of cancer were not infectious, and certainly not contagious. However, during the 1950s, the electron microscopic demonstration of viruses and viral "particles" in cancer tissue, renewed interest in the role of viruses as possible infectious agents in cancer.

Decades earlier, in 1910, Peyton Rous (1879-1970), theo-rized a virus to explain the contagiousness of a form of can-cer in chickens, now known as "Rous sarcoma." Rous showed that a filtered, bacteria-free extract of sarcoma tumor tissue from a diseased chicken could cause new sarco-mas when injected into healthy chickens. Rous' scientific studies indicating the viral "infectiousness" of cancer, were ignored by other medical scientists for more than a half-century. In 1966, at the age of eighty-seven, Peyton Rous finally received a Nobel prize for these discoveries. Viruses are now known to be associated with some forms of cancer in animals.

It has not been decided whether viruses cause cancer in humans. There is some evidence that the "Epstein-Barr" virus may cause "Burkitt's" lymphoma, (a cancer found in Central Africa); and a type of nose and throat cancer, (naso-pharyngeal cancer), found primarily in Chinese adults. "Hepatitis B" virus may be implicated in liver cancer, par-ticularly in those patients with preceding hepatitis. Some researchers think "herpes 2" type viruses may cause cancer of the cervix in women, and cancer of the prostate gland in men.

Despite all this scientific knowledge, there is no conclu-sive proof that viruses cause human cancer. Most damaging to the viral theory of cancer is that viruses cannot be grown from many cancer tumors, nor can viral "particles" or "inclusions" be identified. However, viruses can be extremely elusive. According to Donald Francis, "an electron microscope will not allow the viewer to see virus particles unless the concentration exceeds 1 million per milliliter (33,000 per drop). Thus direct visualization of viruses, even in known infected tissues, is often difficult."

Some scientists think the cancer virus may be "hidden" inside the cancer cells. Bernard Glemser, author of "Man Against Cancer" (1969), describes how viruses may adapt to life within a human cell. "Once they are within a cell they may — temporarily, perhaps — abandon their viral way of life and, for reasons that are still totally beyond our understanding, become incorporated in the cells' own chromosomal material. The cell is thus changed, or transformed; and it is in this condition, among others, that the cell may become malignant. The various immune processes now cannot act specifically against the virus because it no longer exists as a virus, it is simply a particle of nucleic acid which has hidden itself within a complex chain of nucleic acid. It reproduces not as a separate organism but along with the chromosomal material in which it hides."

The suspected sexually transmitted agent of AIDS is thought to be a virus. A number of already-known viruses have been suggested as the agent. The most well-known is the "herpes 2" virus, which can cause severe and uncontrollable infection in AIDS patients. Another virus is the cytomegalovirus, which we shall discuss later in detail. In May 1983, a CDC report indicated that the "human T cell leukemia" virus (HTLV) had been discovered in the "T cell lymphocytes" from several AIDS patients. The report concluded the "HTLV, or an HTLV-like agent, might simply represent another opportunistic agent. Further study is required to determine if any etiologic relationship exists between HTLV and AIDS."

"Adenoviruses" have been "increasingly found in urine from AIDS patients," as reported by Pieter de Jong, *et al* (1983). These viruses were present in about 20% of AIDS patients at Montefiore Hospital in New York City.

There is no question that viruses play some role as pathogenic agents in some patients with cancer and AIDS. Viruses, like bacteria, are ubiquitous in the environment. Our bodies are constantly exposed to them.

Currently, medical science regards viruses and bacteria as distinct, and unrelated, microbiological forms. However, Lida Mattman, Professor of Microbiology, at Wayne State University in Detroit, has considered "it may be that viruses whose structure is not well characterized may actually be part of the life cycle of a bacterium." One study of the "Rous sarcoma" virus by Eleanor Alexander-Jackson, indicated that the virus was actually a "deficient" form of a *bacterium*, which could be isolated consistently from chicken sarcomas.

Although science does not consider a relationship between viruses and bacteria, it is a fact that the largest known viruses approximate the size of the smallest bacteria. In addition, bacteria have "filterable" forms which approximate the size of some viruses. Bacteria are also susceptible to infection with viruses. Viruses which parasitize bacteria are known as "bacteriophages."

Most people with AIDS do not die from the pathogenic effects of one specific agent. They succumb from the combined damaging effects of multiple infectious disease agents. Even when and if the "agent" in AIDS is discovered, clinicians will still have to deal with the superimposed and often lethal effects of these multiple opportunistic infectious microbes.

It is likely that the suspected agent of AIDS triggers the immune defects which allow AIDS to develop. When this elusive agent is found, science will then have to explain what triggers the agent to cause disease.

We have known about microbes for a century. Yet, we do not know why microbes become pathogenic in certain individuals. For instance, we still do not understand why certain people acquire tuberculosis, and leprosy, and yet other individuals exposed to the same microbes do not catch the disease.

At the start of the AIDS epidemic in 1981, the virus most strongly suspected as the agent in AIDS was the cytomegalovirus. Three years later, interest in this virus as the causative agent was waning. Nevertheless, an understanding of the cytomegalovirus and its proposed role in AIDS is essential to unravel some of the mystery of the AIDS epidemic.

References

Chase A: *Virus, a creature of reason. In, Magic Shots. William Morrow and Company, Inc., New York, 1982, pp 237-271.*

Francis DP: *The search for the cause. In, Cahill KM (Ed): The AIDS Epidemic, St. Martin's Press, New York, 1983, pp 137-148.*

Glemser B: *Man Against Cancer. Funk & Wagnalls, New York, 1969, p 191.*

CDC: *Human T-cell leukemia virus infection in patients with acquired immune deficiency syndrome: Preliminary observations. MMWR 32: 233-234, 1983.*

de Jong PJ, Spigland I, Valderrama G, *et al: Adenovirus isolates from urine of patients with acquired immunodeficiency syndrome. Lancet 1: 1293-1296, 1983.*

Mattman LH: *Are any viruses just bacterial variants? In, Cell Wall Deficient Forms. CRC Press, Cleveland, Ohio, 1974, pp 385-386.*

Alexander-Jackson E: *Ultraviolet spectrogramic microscope studies of Rous sarcoma virus cultures in cell-free medium. Ann NY Acad Sci 174: 765-781, 1967.*

11 Cytomegalovirus and AIDS

The virus that has undergone the most intensive investigation as the causative sexually transmitted agent of AIDS, and Kaposi's sarcoma, is the "cytomegalovirus."

Cytomegalovirus is one of four viruses known collectively as the herpes virus group. Within this family of viruses, (all of which look similar under the electron microscope), are the herpes simplex, or "cold sore" viruses; the viruses causing chicken-pox and "shingles," (varicella-zoster virus); the "Epstein-Barr" virus believed to cause infectious mononucleosis, and Burkitt's lymphoma; and cytomegalovirus, a suspected virus in AIDS.

Cytomegalovirus is a common virus of man and animals, and is found throughout the world. Some newborns are infected with cytomegalovirus, having contracted the virus from the mother's blood. It is likely that all human beings eventually become infected with cytomegalovirus. Fortunately, most human infection with this virus produces no symptoms, or such mild symptoms that the viral infection usually goes unnoticed.

Cytomegalovirus and other herpes viruses may persist within the human body in an undetectable "latent" state. Cytomegalovirus has been found in the blood and secretions of both healthy and ill individuals. The virus can sometimes be grown from saliva, urine, and feces, from the cervical

81

secretions and breast milk in women, and from the semen in men.

In a 1982 study of seventy children, (ages 3-65 months), in a Birmingham, Alabama, day care center, Robert Pass, *et al*, found that 53% of the children were excreting cytomegalovirus in the urine; 45% were excreting cytomegalovirus in the saliva.

There is evidence that cytomegalovirus can be transmitted by blood transfusions. A. M. Prince, *et al* (1971), noted the development of "complement-fixing antibody" to cytomegalovirus in 21% of 72 patients who received multiple transfusions. Over one-half of an immunosuppressed group of transplant recipients developed cytomegalovirus antibodies, after transfusion.

Laboratory experiments in animals have shown that cytomegalovirus can be easily passed from animal-to-animal, and is therefore transmissible. However, each animal has its own unique type of cytomegalovirus, which cannot be transmitted to animals of different species. Laboratory inoculation of animals with cytomegalovirus causes immunosuppression of the immune system.

When a human cell is infected with cytomegalovirus, microscopic changes may take place within the nucleus of the cell, and in the surrounding cell cytoplasm. These pathologic changes may result in the formation of viral-caused "inclusion bodies" within the cell nucleus and cytoplasm. The inclusion bodies produced by cytomegalovirus are quite distinctive, and can be easily identified by pathologists studying tissue with an ordinary light microscope. Cytomegalovirus may also cause the infected cells to become very large, resulting in the formation of "giant cells." The name cytomegalovirus ("cyto" = cell, and "megalia" = giant) was given to the virus producing the large "giant" cells characteristically found in diseased patients with "cytomegalic inclusion disease."

The pathologic effects of cytomegalovirus infection were first noted in 1904, in a stillborn baby who had acquired syphilis from its mother. At the autopsy, the characteristic cytomegalovirus inclusion bodies were detected in the cells of the baby's lungs, kidneys, and liver. However, most medical scientists did not realize these inclusions were due to a virus infection until a half-century later. In the early part of this century, microbiologists erroneously interpreted the inclusion bodies as "protozoal parasites," (much like *Pneumocystis carinii*).

In 1921, Ernest Goodpasture and Fritz Talbott, pathologists at Harvard University, declared that the "giant cells" of "cytomegalia" were not produced by *any* infectious agent, including viruses. The pathologists concluded (wrongly) that the viral-induced giant cells were "independent" and "capable perhaps of wandering about, exhibiting a certain similarity to protozoa." However, Goodpasture and Talbott were perceptive in realizing that these inclusion bodies could also be seen in the salivary glands of the mouth in many "normal" laboratory animals.

During the 1930s, it was discovered that as many as one-third of all infants had inclusion bodies in their salivary glands. These bodies were similar to those seen in animals. On the basis of animal experiments, a few researchers began to suspect these characteristic inclusion bodies were related to actual virus infection. A few pathologists also realized a spread of the "salivary gland virus" infection to other organs of the body could cause the death of some infants. Until the 1950s, scientists studying cytomegalovirus, were hampered by the inability to grow the virus outside of tissue cells, and by the inability to transmit the human type of cytomegalovirus infection to laboratory animals.

As late as 1950, both cytomegalovirus, and the cytomegalic inclusion disease which the virus produced, were largely unknown to medical doctors. J. P. Wyatt, *et al* (1950), studied 66 cases of cytomegalovirus disease (64 infants and 2 adults). They wrote in *The Journal of Pediatrics*, "it is interesting to note that even textbooks of pediatrics, bacteriology, and virology, do not discuss this condition. The main reasons for this omission probably are: first, a failure to recognize its importance (since it is largely a 'pathologists disease'), and second, the reluctance of many authorities to accept a disease as of established viral etiology in the absence of transmissibility to animals." With this publication, pediatricians were made aware that the cytomegalovirus could harm and kill newborns and young infants.

During the 1950s, the frequent association of cytomegalovirus with the parasite *Pneumocystis carinii*, in epidemic "infantile pneumonia" in Europe, was first noted.

H. Hamperl (1956), a German pathologist, first made American pathologists aware of the dangerous, and often fatal, lung infection produced by these two microbes. Hamperl clearly understood that widespread infection with cytomegalovirus *alone* was sufficient to kill newborn infants. But Hamperl was the first to seriously suspect that the virus *alone* could not produce a fatal pneumonia in an *adult.*

The frequent combined lung infection with the cytomegalovirus *and* the Pneumocystis parasite, in adult pneumonia cases with AIDS, would continue to perplex epidemiologists and researchers in the 1980s.

In 1970, Nai-San Wang, *et al*, from Montreal, Canada, in a paper entitled, *"Pneumocystis carinii* and cytomegalovirus infection," attempted to explain the exceedingly high incidence of combined infection with these two agents. They studied the lung cells of two patients who died with pneumonia. The cells were magnified over 100,000 times with the electron microscope.

The first patient was a 35 year-old man who had received a kidney transplant in 1964. He was treated with immunosuppressive drugs, until his death from pneumonia in 1969. One week before death, *Pneumocystis carinii*, and bacteria *(Streptococcus viridans),* were discovered in his lung. At the autopsy, an unsuspected metastasizing cancer of the intestine was also discovered.

The second patient was a 60 year-old Japanese woman who had died with pneumonitis, in Montreal, in 1945. At the autopsy, her lungs were infected with *two* kinds of bacteria, *(Streptococcus viridans* and *Escherichia coli).* This case had been reported three times previously. Gardner McMillan reported this patient in 1947, as a case of "fatal inclusion disease pneumonitis, *of unknown cause*." In 1950, Wyatt, *et al*, reported the case as one of many examples of fatal viral infection with the newly-recognized cytomegalovirus. Hamperl, in 1956, also restudied the same woman's case, and discovered a previously unrecognized Pneumocystis parasitic lung infection.

Wang's group, using the electron microscope, observed particles of cytomegalovirus within the lungs. Remarkably, similar viral particles were also seen *within* the Pneumocystis parasites, suggesting the parasite was *also* infected with cytomegalovirus. The researchers thought this might explain the frequent combined infection of the lungs with these two different organisms. They concluded that "although the idea of infection of a protozoan may at first appear strange, there is good evidence of infection of protozoa and fungi by viruses."

These two Canadian cases are prophetic of future cases in which multiple opportunistic infection with viruses, bacteria, fungi, and parasites would occur in AIDS. In Wang's first case, the unusual association of kidney transplantation, immunosuppression, opportunistic infection, and cancer, was noteworthy in 1969. Years later, the association of immunosuppression, opportunistic infection, and cancer would be commonplace in homosexual men dying with AIDS.

The role of cytomegalovirus, if any, in the development of cancer, is obscure. Only with AIDS in gays, have certain authorities seriously considered cytomegalovirus as a possible cause of cancer, particularly Kaposi's sarcoma.

What was the relationship between cytomegalovirus and cancer before the onset of the AIDS epidemic?

In 1971, Peter Rosen and Steven Hajdu, pathologists at Memorial Hospital in New York City, identified inclusions of cytomegalovirus in the lungs of 17 of 5,788 consecutive autopsies of cancer patients. Pneumocystis parasites were detected in only 5 patients.

In a later paper (1978), entitled "Cytomegalovirus infection in cancer patients," Rosen wrote: "It is apparent from the foregoing review that the clinical and laboratory manifestations of cytomegalovirus infection in patients with neoplastic (cancerous) disease are very varied and difficult to interpret." Clinical signs of cytomegalovirus infection may include hepatitis-like symptoms, fatigue, varying degrees of pneumonia, anemia, gastrointestinal symptoms, and kidney disturbances. "Many of these complications may also result from therapy, other infections, or the underlying disease and are therefore not specific."

According to Rosen, "the most reliable evidence of cytomegalovirus infection is the finding of the typical inclusions in a destructive tissue lesion, in microscopic examination." Rosen stresses that cytomegalovirus may be excreted in the urine, even in the absence of viral disease. Isolation of the virus from the sputum or saliva was considered "of dubious value."

Later, in some AIDS cases, cytomegalovirus inclusion bodies could not be identified at autopsy, nor could the virus be isolated from the diseased tissue, or observed in the Kaposi's sarcoma tumors by electron microscopy. Still, many scientists insist that cytomegalovirus is related to AIDS for the following reasons. First, as many as 90% of homosexuals have serologic evidence of cytomegalovirus infection. This does not necessarily mean all these men are infected with cytomegalovirus in the usual sense, but only that at some time of their life, their bodies had been exposed to the virus. Second, cytomegalovirus may be present in the body fluids, allowing possible sexual transmission of this virus, between gay men. Third, is the previously mentioned proven ability of cytomegalovirus to depress the immune system.

During the past decade, studies by Gaetano Giraldo, *et al*, have indicated that cytomegalovirus may be found in Kaposi's sarcoma, the most common form of cancer found in AIDS patients. Giraldo has studied skin tumors from European and American cases of "classic" Kaposi's sarcoma, as well as tumors from Africans and gays. Herpes-type virus particles were found in tumor cell cultures grown from 5 of 8 African cases of Kaposi's sarcoma tumors. A virus was isolated from one case, and was identified as a strain of cytomegalovirus. Four of seven newborn and young baboons injected with this strain, died within 7 days to 10 months. Two of four baboons developed enlarged lymph glands. However, no viral particles could be detected within these glands. The virus could be recovered from the animal tissue but did not appear to have any consistent damaging effects upon the cell culture. Giraldo was able to detect a "cytomegalovirus related antigen" in a low percentage of cells (0.1 -0.5%) within the culture.

It was also determined that European and American cases of Kaposi's sarcoma had a higher degree of immunologic reactivity to cytomegalovirus than did the African cases. The reactivity to cytomegalovirus of both African Kaposi's sarcoma cases and "healthy" black Africans without cancer was about the same.

The search for viruses in AIDS continues. Evidence is accumulating in the third year of the epidemic that other viruses, such as adenoviruses, retroviruses, the "human T cell leukemia virus," and the Epstein-Barr virus, may also be associated with AIDS. However as the history of AIDS enfolds in this book, it will be suggested that the most likely cause of AIDS is *not a "virus,"* but a *bacterium,* which can be easily seen microscopically. This microbe has been observed not only in AIDS and Kaposi's sarcoma, but also in many forms of "regular" forms of cancer, as well.

References

Pass RF, August AM, Dworsky M. *et al: Cytomegalovirus in a day care center. N Engl J Med 307: 477-479, 1982.*

Weller TH: *Cytomegaloviruses: Ubiquitous agents with protean clinical manifestations. N Engl J Med 285: 203-214, 1971.*

Prince AM, Szmuness W, Millian SJ, et al: A serologic study of cytomegalovirus infections associated with blood transfusions. New Engl J Med 284: 1125-1130, 1971.

Jesionek, and Kiolemenoglue: Ueber einen Befund von protoenaritgen Gebilden in den Organen eines hereditar-luetischen Fotus. Munch Med Wchnschr 43: 1905, 1904.

Goodpasture EW, and Talbot FB: Concerning the nature of "protozoan like" cells in certain lesions of infancy. Amer J Dis Child 21: 415-425, 1920.

Wyatt JP, Saxton J, Lee RS, et al: Generalized cytomegalic inclusion disease. J Pediatrics 36: 271-294, 1950.

Hamperl H: Pneumocystis infection and cytomegaly of the lungs in the newborn and adult. Amer J Pathol 32: 1-13, 1956.

Wang JS, Huang SH, Thurlbeck WM: Combined Pneumocystis carinii and cytomegalovirus infection. Arch Pathol 90: 529-535, 1970.

McMillan GC: Fatal inclusion disease pneumonitis in an adult. Amer J Pathol 23: 995-1003, 1947.

Rosen P, and Hajdu S: Cytomegalovirus disease at autopsy of patients with cancer. Amer J Clin Pathol 55: 749-756, 1971.

Rosen PR: Cytomegalovirus infection in cancer patients. In, Pathol Annu 2, Appleton Century Crofts, New York, 1978, pp 175-208.

Giraldo G, Beth E, Kyalwazi SK: Etiological implications of Kaposi's sarcoma. In, Antibiotics and Chemotherapy 29, S Karger, Basel, 1981, pp 12-29.

12   Cancer in AIDS: One Disease or Many?

Tragically, chemotherapeutic drugs used to treat cancer may ultimately cause the formation of another "different" cancer. For example, after chemotherapy, about three percent of patients with Hodgkin's lymphoma may develop "non-Hodgkin's lymphoma," or leukemia. The reason for these "second" cancers is unknown. Scientists, such as Richard Fisher of the National Cancer Institute, assume "two different diseases are involved." The theory is that chemotherapeutic drugs depress the immune system, resulting in the development of "new" cancers.

Undoubtedly, AIDS patients who can survive the life-threatening effects of opportunistic infections and Kaposi's sarcoma, will also be at risk for the development of "second" cancers. Before AIDS, it was already known that over one-third of the patients with "classic" Kaposi's sarcoma were likely to develop a second cancer, usually of the lymphoma type.

Other cancers besides Kaposi's sarcoma can develop in gay men with AIDS. In 1981, John Ziegler, *et al*, from San Francisco, reported four men with cancer resembling "Burkitt's lymphoma." Burkitt's lymphoma is an extremely rare cancer in America, but is common in Central Africa.

The cancer affects black children and young adults, causing enlargement of the lymph glands, and other organs. Without chemotherapy, death often occurs within 6 to 12 weeks. The tumors may shrink rapidly with chemotherapy, but the cancer often recurs.

Most scientists now believe the Epstein-Barr virus causes Burkitt's lymphoma. However, this has not been proven. Over 80 percent of healthy, normal, black African children under the age of five years carry the virus. As many as 20 percent of the tumors occurring in Africa, do not show evidence of the virus. It is possible the virus may only reside as a "passenger" in the tumor tissue. Only 15 to 20 percent of Burkitt's lymphoma tumors, found elsewhere in the world, contain Epstein-Barr virus. Two of three tumors tested in San Francisco patients contained Epstein-Barr virus "antigens." One tumor also contained cytomegalovirus antigens.

Researchers, such as Joseph Sonnabend, *et al*, now propose that cytomegalovirus causes Kaposi's sarcoma in gay men, and that Epstein-Barr virus causes Burkitt's lymphoma.

Some recent studies cast doubt on the role of the Epstein-Barr virus in Burkitt's lymphoma. Scientists studying cell chromosomes and cancer, concluded in a report published in *The Journal of the American Medical Association*, (November 19, 1982), that "Epstein-Barr virus, which has long been linked to Burkitt's lymphoma, either plays a secondary role or, possibly no role, in the disease's etiology."

Most physicians believe cancer is many different diseases. The American Cancer Society, while readily admitting the cause (or causes) of cancer is unknown, is adamant in its concept that "not all cancers are the same." David Wellisch and Joel Yager recently wrote in *Ca, a Cancer Journal for Physicians* (1983), "current knowledge reveals the diversity of cancers; significant differences exist with respect to etiologies, pathogenesis, natural histories, and so on. To lump all cancers together is equivalent to lumping all heart diseases, lung diseases, or anemias together."

Although most scientists agree that cancer is many

different diseases, a notable exception is Lewis Thomas, who questions that concept in his book "The Youngest Science" (1983). "Because of such different responses, (to the treatment of cancer), it is believed in some quarters that cancer is really not a single disease but perhaps a hundred different ones, each requiring its own separate research program and, ultimately, its own special kind of treatment. Sometimes this rather bleak point of view is put forward defensively by the groups most concerned with public support for cancer research." "In the end, when all the basic facts are in, I think it will turn out that all forms of cancer, in whatever organs and of whatever cell types, are a single disease, caused by a single, central controlling mechanism gone wrong. The idea that cancer in different organs represents separate, different diseases seems to me beyond belief at today's level of knowledge."

In the past few years, there has been some attempt to bring together previously diverse and "different" forms of cancer.

In 1981, Bijan Safai, and Robert Good, scientists at the Memorial Sloan Kettering Cancer Center in New York City, wrote, "our own observations and those of others clearly show a high incidence of second primary cancers, particularly lymphoreticular neoplasms in Kaposi's sarcoma patients. This close association of lymphoreticular neoplasms and Kaposi's sarcoma suggests that a tumor inducer or promotor continues to operate in these individuals, and that the etiopathogenic mechanisms of lymphomas and Kaposi's sarcoma are either common to both or are closely linked in a similar manner. It is now commonly proposed that Kaposi's sarcoma be considered, along with leukemia and lymphoma, as part of a spectrum of disease affecting the lymphoreticular system."

The possibility of developing *other* forms of cancer, from sexual contact with AIDS patients, is illustrated by a case report from the Kaposi's Sarcoma Clinic in San Francisco.

Marcus Conant, *et al* (1982), reported the "most unusual" development of a malignant tumor of the tongue (squamous cell cancer) of a 29 year-old gay man, who was the sexual partner of a 35 year-old man with Kaposi's sarcoma.

There is even new statistical evidence to suggest that an increased incidence of anorectal cancer may be correlated with homosexual activity. Fortunately, this type of cancer is still rare in young and middle-aged gay men.

The scientific evidence, and the issue of whether cancer is one disease or many, should be carefully studied, especially by the gay community. The national, social, economic, political, religious, and scientific implications of AIDS, and "gay cancer" are enormous. In particular, the fears of the general public concerning AIDS may well contribute to the possible separation and eventual alienation, between "gay" and heterosexual society.

The rapid spread of the AIDS epidemic within the gay community has rekindled the public's suspicion that some forms of cancer may be catching. The public believes "gay cancer" is contagious, untreatable, and invariably fatal.

Some physicians are reinforcing the public's attitude by emphasizing that AIDS and cancer in gay men is a *venereal* disease. J. B. Stapcznski, M.D., wrote the following letter entitled "The Spread of AIDS" which appeared in *The Los Angeles Times*, (June 10, 1983).

"Those recent demonstrators against AIDS need to admit that the gay life style is responsible for the rapid spread of AIDS in this country. While fortunately attitudes are changing, many people in this country refuse to acknowledge that life style and habits greatly influence health.

Refusing to accept responsibility for our own actions enables the victim of lung cancer to blame fate rather than the cigarette habit. So it is with AIDS. Face facts. AIDS is predominantly a venereal type disease found in incredibly promiscuous male homosexuals.

For crying out loud, don't blame "society." Just like the victim of gonorrhea, syphilis, or herpes, most AIDS victims need to acknowledge how they contracted the disease.

This is not to deny that AIDS is a serious and increasing problem; it has killed more people than toxic shock and Legionnaires' disease combined. Of course further research should be funded.

Everybody, including AIDS victims and the gay population, should be willing to accept responsibility for their actions."

Is "gay" cancer somehow really *different* from "straight" cancer? Is it possible to get cancer from "straight" sex? Are all those different kinds of cancer really different?

In order to attempt to answer these questions, we must turn our attention to the nature of cancer, and to the possible contagiousness of cancer. But first, let us examine the relationship of some cancers to sex and sexuality.

References

Armitage JO, Dick FR, Goeken JA, *et al: Second lymphoid malignant neoplasms occurring in patients treated for Hodgkin's disease. Arch Intern Med 143: 445-450, 1983.*

Fisher RI: *Non-Hodgkin's lymphomas after treatment of Hodgkin's disease. Arch Intern Med 143: 427, 1983.*

Safai B, and Good RA: *Kaposi's sarcoma: A review and recent developments. Ca, A Cancer Journal for Clinicians 31: 2-12, 1981.*

Ziegler JL, Miner RC, Rosenbaum E, *et al: Outbreak of Burkitt's-like lymphoma in homosexual men. Lancet 2: 631-633, 1982.*

Ziegler JL: *Burkitt's lymphoma. New Engl J Med 305:* *735-745, 1981.*

Sonnabend J, Witkin SS, Purtilo DT: *Acquired immuno-deficiency syndrome, opportunistic infections, and malignancies in male homosexuals. JAMA 249:* *2370-2374, 1983.*

Medical News: *Migrant oncogene - Burkitt's lymphoma link. JAMA 248: 2424-2426, 1982.*

Wellisch DK, and Yager J: *Is there a cancer-prone personality? Ca, A Cancer Journal for Clinicians 33: 145-153, 1983.*

Thomas L: *The Youngest Science, The Viking Press, New York, 1983, pp 201-202.*

Conant MA, Volberding P, Fletcher V, *et al: Squamous cell carcinoma in sexual partner of Kaposi sarcoma patient. Lancet 1: 286, 1982.*

Kondlapoodi P: *Anorectal cancer and homosexuality. JAMA 248: 2114-2115, 1982.*

Stapcznski JS: *Spread of AIDS, Los Angeles Times, June 10, 1983.*

13   Sex, AIDS, and Cancer

"Scientists have found that cancer is not contagious. No one can catch any form of the disease from another person. Cancer is not transmitted to a sex partner by sexual intercourse, nor is it transmitted by coughing, sneezing, or any other kind of physical contact." National Cancer Institute, DHEW Publication No. (NIH) 79-1566.

"Is cancer contagious? Despite 100 years of research, scientists have never found the least evidence that human cancer is contagious. Infectious diseases caused by a virus are usually contagious. But cancer, even cancer caused by a virus, is not." The Cancer Reference Book. Direct and Clear Answers to Everyone's Questions, 1979.

"After watching friends and lovers die, certain that tricking and drugs killed them, many of us now regard our once glamourous and exciting lifestyle as toxic. We are left frightened, nervous, and confused. Do all those years of frenzied drug orgies at the baths mean it is only a matter of time before we are stricken? We are obsessed about our health. A minor sore throat, a slight black and blue mark conjures up visions of

95

pneumonia or cancer." Marty Levine: Fearing fear
itself. In, Gay Men's Health Crisis Newsletter 1, July,
1982.

*"Although the cause of AIDS remains unknown: the
Public Health Service recommends the following: Sex-
ual contact should be avoided with persons known or
suspected to have AIDS."* Centers for Disease Control,
Morbidity and Mortality Weekly Report 32:102,
March 4, 1983.

Along with gay liberation, the sexual revolution, and the
widespread use of "recreational drugs" in the 1970s, came a
skyrocketing incidence of gonorrhea, syphilis, hepatitis,
herpes virus infections, venereal warts, and scabies. Half
the number of annual cases of syphilis in America were
occurring in homosexual men. Although patients with these
diseases were temporarily alarmed, these diseases were
rarely life-threatening. In most cases, a quick visit to the
doctor for treatment, was all that was needed to put a
patient back into the endless sexual marathon.

With the onset of AIDS in the 1980s, a new awareness of
the dangers of sexual promiscuity was emerging. Sex was
still sensational, but scientists were suggesting that sex,
especially "gay" sex, could also be lethal!

But sex has always been risky. Rape, sexual violence,
unwanted pregnancies, and serious venereal diseases have
plagued the lives of countless numbers of people since the
beginning of time. In addition, even discounting the issue of
heterosexual and homosexual sex, there are serious cancer
risks inherent within the sexes. For instance, breast cancer
in women in America, is over 1000 times more common than
cancer of the breast in men. In 1980, 35,000 American
women died of breast cancer.

Cancer of the genital organs in men and women claims
45,000 lives yearly. Prostate gland cancer in men kills
21,000 persons a year. As men get older, the incidence of

prostate gland cancer rises markedly. Autopsy studies of men over the age of 75 have shown that about one-half of all men have microscopic evidence of this form of cancer, even though the prostate gland cancer may not be clinically detectible during life.

About 7,600 women die yearly from cancer of the cervix, the part of the uterus (womb) that extends into the vagina. Some scientists believe cervical cancer is directly related to heterosexual activity, and to sexual hygienic practices. Researchers have even suggested cervical cancer is a venereal disease caused by the "herpes 2" virus. Women with genital herpes infection have a greater risk of developing cervical cancer. The recent sexual revolution may be responsible for the fact that more cases are now being diagnosed in young, sexually active women, twenty years of age and under.

Cancer of the cervix is more common in poor women, and in women marrying, or engaging in sexual activity, at an early age. Cervical cancer is also more common in prostitutes, and in women whose sexual partners are uncircumcised. Cervical cancer is rare in nuns, and in Jewish, Moslem, and Navajo women.

The possibility that certain heterosexual activity might lead to the development of cervical cancer in women has been deliberately downplayed by cancer educators. John Wakefield wrote in "Persons at High Risk for Cancer" (1975), "there are known risks to women in sexual promiscuity," — "but can we publicize the relationship between promiscuity and cervical cancer as a strong feature of the (cancer prevention) program?" Quite simply, cancer educators worry that many women will not participate in genital cancer testing due to the possible "fear that the test will reveal past sexual adventures."

Cervical cancer in women is much more common in cultures where men are not circumcised. This had led a few scientists to believe that some agent in the male "smegma" (the cheese-like glandular secretions of the foreskin in uncircumcised men) might be capable of producing cancer.

The circumcision of Jewish men is thought to be a possible reason for the low rates of cervical cancer in Jewish women. Cancer of the penis is extremely rare in men who have been circumcised in infancy.

An interesting study was performed by Henry Heins, *et al* (1958), in which smegma obtained from male foreskins was inserted into the vaginas of a strain of mice which normally do not develop cancer of the cervix. The researchers were able to produce a few experimental cervical cancers in the mice, by frequent insertions of smegma.

In another set of experiments, bacterial microbes were cultured from human smegma, and then inserted into the vaginas of the mice, to determine if cancer could develop. Curiously, the insertion of "acid-fast" bacteria, (*Mycobacterium smegmatis*), normally found in smegma, resulted in the almost immediate death of 8 of 14 mice! The study concluded that smegma from the foreskin of men might in some way cause cancer of the cervix in women, as well as cancer of the penis in men.

Cancer of the penis, although rare in Europe and North America, occurs frequently in Asia, Africa, and Latin America, where this kind of cancer is responsible for as many as 15% of the cancer tumors found in men.

In Uganda, Africa, which has one of the highest rates of Kaposi's sarcoma in the world, cancer of the penis is the most common tumor found in men. However, the incidence of penile cancer varies tremendously among African tribes, irrespective of whether circumcision is practiced or not. The reason for this is not clear. R. Schmauz, and D. K. Jain (1971), pathologists at Makerere Medical School in Kampala, Uganda, have concluded that infectious microbes such as bacteria or viruses may cause cancer of the penis.

Surprisingly, *no* scientist has ever suggested the extremely high rate of both Kaposi's sarcoma and cancer of the penis, in Ugandans, or any other African group, is in any way caused by either a sexually transmitted agent, or by homosexual activity.

A few scientists have been rather outspoken, and perhaps

judgmental, in reporting the social and sexual behavior of certain Africans. In 1962, Stephen Rothman commented on the purported "loose family life" in Uganda, by stating "Bantu men often desert their wives and children and take in new wives with their children, so that they themselves frequently do not know where 'their' children came from, nor where the others went."

Although sexual activity has not been correlated with Kaposi's sarcoma in Africa, most scientists have concluded that "gay sex" between men is responsible for most cases of Kaposi's sarcoma, and AIDS, in America. However, there is no connection between lesbianism and AIDS. It is remarkable that three years after the onset of the AIDS epidemic, *no* cases have been discovered in gay women.

As previously mentioned, cancer of the prostate gland is a common form of cancer in men. The relationship, if any, between sexual activity, and prostate gland cancer, is unclear. The incidence of prostate gland cancer varies tremendously between men of different races. For instance, there are twice as many cases of prostate cancer among black American men than among whites.

Robert Steele, *et al* (1971), concluded that men with prostate gland cancer appear to have a greater sexual drive, and that a sexually transmitted agent might be an important causative factor in this type of cancer.

In another report, John Feminella and John Lattimer (1974), urologists at Colombia University in New York City, studied 101 wives of men with prostate cancer. The women were found to have an abnormally high incidence of genital organ cancer, as compared to a "control" group of women whose husbands had "benign," non-cancerous diseases of the prostate. The researchers suggested "the possible communicable role of prostatic carcinoma (cancer) through sexual intercourse, resulting in a higher incidence of genital carcinoma (cervix and breast), in the spouse."

The AIDS epidemic has brought about a serious reappraisal by medical scientists of the possible connection between sexual activity and cancer. For the first time, a sexually transmissible infectious agent is being sought in Kaposi's sarcoma, a heretofore rare form of cancer, attacking as many as one-third of people who have AIDS.

In March 1983, the Public Health Service recommended "that sexual contact be avoided with persons known, or suspected of having AIDS." Most physicians believe this public recommendation is warranted, even though a proven sexually transmitted agent has not been discovered in AIDS.

No health-conscious person would knowingly consent to sexual activity with an untreated person having syphilis or tuberculosis. For similar reasons, it would probably be unwise to be the sexual partner of AIDS and Kaposi's sarcoma patients. Although syphilis and tuberculosis can be treated successfully, there is no cure at present for AIDS and Kaposi's sarcoma.

Physicians are now suggesting certain changes in homosexual practices be made during the current epidemic in an attempt to reduce the risk of AIDS. However, all doctors are not necessarily in agreement with each other, on this issue.

The American Association of Physicians for Human Rights issued a "Statement on AIDS and Healthful Gay Male Sexual Activity," on February 19, 1983, which reads as follows:

Reducing Risks

Two major steps you can take to dramatically reduce your risk of AIDS are the following:

1. Decrease the *number* of *different* men with whom you have sex, and particularly with those men who also have many different sex partners. This does *not* mean to reduce the frequency of sex with any *one* partner, but only the number of different partners.
2. Do not inject any drugs not prescribed for you; avoid sexual contact with intravenous drug users.

Certain sexual practices are known to be associated with an increased risk of sexually transmitted diseases. Reducing these factors may decrease your risk of AIDS:

1. One time encounters with anonymous partners and/or group sex.
2. Oral-anal contact (rimming).
3. "Fisting" (both giving and receiving).
4. Active or passive rectal intercourse (use of condoms may be helpful).
5. Fecal contamination (scat).

An additional probable risk factor may be mucous membrane (mouth or rectum) contact with semen or urine.

Positive Steps You Should Take

1. Know your sex partner and ask about his health. When in doubt, back out!
2. Increase touching and general body contact; the risk of kissing on the lips is unknown.
3. Shower before sex and inspect your partner.
4. Take good care of your body and general health (adequate rest, good nutrition, physical exercise, reduction of stress, reduction of toxic substances (alcohol, cigarettes, marijuana, "poppers," non-prescription drugs).

If you know or suspect that you have any disease you could give to someone else, don't risk the health of others by having sex. Consult a personal physician who is up to date on gay health issues, and have the courage to tell the physician you are gay and wish to discuss AIDS.

By 1984, the AIDS epidemic had forced most gay men to alter their sexual practices. Some previously promiscuous men were now considering monogamy, fidelity, and even celibacy. Many men were spending less time in bars and bathhouses. The sexual use of "recreational drugs" was becoming less popular. Sadly, some brave men were caring for their friends and lovers who were dying of AIDS.

By 1984, one hardly needed the Surgeon General to label the gay sexual lifestyle of the 1970s as clearly dangerous to your health.

References

Levitt PM, Guralnick ES, Kagan AR, and Gilbert H: *The Cancer Reference Book. Paddington Press Ltd., New York and London, 1979, p 30.*

Levine M: *Fearing fear itself. In Gay Men's Health Crisis Newsletter 1: 14-17, (July) 1982.*

CDC: *Prevention of acquired immune deficiency syndrome (AIDS): Report of inter-agency recommendations. MMWR 32: 101-103, 1983.*

Silverberg E, Lubera JA: *A review of American Cancer Society estimates of cancer cases and cancer deaths. Ca, A Cancer Journal for Clinicians 33: 2-25, 1983.*

Barber HRK: *Cervical cancer. In McGowan L (Ed): Gynecologic Oncology. Appleton Century Crofts, New York, 1978, pp 202-216.*

Wakefield J: *Education of the public. In, Fraumeni JF (Ed): Persons at High Risk of Cancer. Academic Press Inc., New York, 1975, pp 415-434.*

Heins HC Jr, Dennis EJ, Pratt-Thomas HR: *The possible role of smegma in carcinoma of the cervix. Amer J Obstet Gynecol 76: 726-735, 1958.*

Schmauz R, and Jain DK: *Geographical variation of carcinoma of the penis. Brit J Cancer 25: 25-32, 1971.*

Steele R, Lees RE, Krause AS, *et al: Sexual factors in the epidemiology of cancer of the prostate. J Chron Dis 24: 29-37, 1971.*

Feminella JG Jr, and Lattimer JK: *An apparent increase in genital carcinoma among wives of men with prostatic carcinomas: An epidemiologic survey. Pirquet Bull Clin Med 20: 3-10, 1974.*

American Association of Physicians for Human Rights. *The AAPHR statement on AIDS and blood donation. Feb 19, 1983. PO Box 14366, San Francisco, California 94114.*

14 The Nature of Cancer in AIDS

"Three of 6 patients with Kaposi's sarcoma developed their symptoms after sexual contact with persons who already had symptoms of Kaposi's sarcoma. One of these 3 patients developed symptoms of Kaposi's sarcoma 9 months after sexual contact, another patient developed symptoms 13 months after contact, and a third patient developed symptoms 22 months after contact." (CDC: A cluster of Kaposi's sarcoma and *Pneumocystis carinii* pneumonia among homosexual male residents of Los Angeles and Orange counties, California. CDC: Morbidity and Mortality Weekly Report, June 18, 1982.

One American out of every four will be striken with cancer sometime during his or her lifetime. After the age of fifty, the odds are worse. One person in three will develop cancer.

It has often been claimed that a patient with a malignant cancer tumor can be cured if the tumor is removed early. Unfortunately, by the time an internal cancer is discovered it is often truly *not* an early cancer.

The surgeon may, in all honesty, tell the patient that he "got it all." The pathologist may also confirm that the area around the tumor is microscopically "clear," or free of malignant cancer cells.

Nevertheless, in many cases, the original cancer will return or regrow, either in the same area from which it was removed, or in a new area of the body. Thus, even though the cancer was removed early, the patient may still die of the disease.

The scientific explanation for the cancer recurrence is that some "invisible" cancer cells were left behind, or that the tumor, in retrospect, was not really removed early enough. Another common explanation is that, before the surgery, the cancer cells had already broken off from the tumor, and had spread or "metastasized," to other distant areas of the body.

Some "holistic" medical practitioners believe that cancer, even in its earliest stages, is a disease of the whole body, and is not limited solely to the tumor itself. Therefore, the whole body must be brought back to wellness, in order to treat cancer successfully. Certainly, cancers such as leukemia of the blood, and lymphomas of the lymphatic gland system, are whole body (systemic) cancers from the very beginning.

Whether cancer is a local, or a systemic disease, from the outset, one thing is clear. Chemotherapeutic drugs used to treat cancer affect the cells of the entire body. Thus, modern treatment with chemotherapy is systemic treatment of cancer.

One-third of all patients with AIDS either have, or will develop, a malignant cancer such as Kaposi's sarcoma, or other forms of cancer. For this reason, AIDS must be considered a "pre-cancerous" disease, as well as a systemic illness. The incidence of cancer in AIDS patients would undoubtedly be higher, but the majority of seriously ill patients die within two years with opportunistic infection, and do not live long enough to develop cancer.

Is cancer contagious? The high incidence of Kaposi's sarcoma in gay men with AIDS, has again suggested to scientists that some forms of cancer may be contagious.

A century ago, some scientists believed, and attempted to prove, that cancer was both an infectious and transmissible disease caused by "cancer parasites." The idea of a cancer parasite was discarded by most scientific authorities in the early part of this century. Cancer was emphatically declared to be neither an infectious, nor a contagious disease. However, during the past few decades, it has become fashionable to consider viruses, but certainly not bacteria, as possible causative agents in certain forms of cancer, especially Kaposi's sarcoma.

Koposi's sarcoma is a unique form of cancer because the tumors are often "multicentric," meaning new blood tumors of Kaposi's sarcoma can occur anywhere on the skin, or within the body. New Kaposi's sarcoma tumors arise independently, and do not originate from cells which have broken off and metastasized from the original tumor.

The remarkable ability of some malignant cancer cells to regrow, and to metastasize throughout the body, is the reason that radiation, surgery, and chemotherapy, often fail to cure cancer.

The diagnosis of cancer is always made by the pathologist. Strangely, there is still some doubt in the minds of some pathologists, as to whether Kaposi's sarcoma is truly a cancer. Jose Costa and Alan Robson, pathologists at the National Cancer Institute, have recently stated (1983) that "the epidemic of the generalized form of Kaposi's sarcoma among patients with AIDS, is regarded by many as an opportunity to gain insight into the pathogenesis, prophylaxis, and treatment of neoplasia (cancer). That may well be, but the idea that Kaposi's sarcoma, in its disseminated form, is not a neoplasm, is seldom considered."

If Kaposi's sarcoma in gay men with AIDS is *not* cancer, as these pathologists claim, then the use of chemotherapy in Kaposi's sarcoma, which further depresses the immune system, should be seriously questioned. At present, chemotherapy is the only orthodox treatment of widespread Kaposi's sarcoma. The experimental drug "interferon" has been used in the treatment of Kaposi's sarcoma in AIDS patients. The results of such treatment have been varied. In some patients, there has been some temporary shrinkage of the tumors, but interferon has apparently failed to cure cases of Kaposi's sarcoma associated with AIDS.

The decision to accept, or to reject chemotherapy, is a most difficult one for the AIDS patient with cancer. The risk of acquiring opportunistic infection is further increased by chemotherapy. But chemotherapy is the only accepted form of treatment for Kaposi's sarcoma in AIDS patients. There are no alternatives.

AIDS is one of the most serious diseases of the twentieth century. Doctors have been powerless to treat it, and to stop it. The reason for this powerlessness is clear. Physicians have not fully appreciated the apparent contagiousness of some forms of cancer, nor have scientists devised a truly effective treatment for many forms of cancer.

Eventually, the true microbial cause of cancer will be understood. Scientists will then discover that both AIDS *and* cancer are infectious diseases. Doctors will discover that AIDS *is* cancer, and cancer *is* AIDS. But the most startling revelation, which will revolutionize medicine in the twenty first century, will be the discovery that the blood stream of all human beings normally harbors the microbes that are the cause of both diseases.

References

Costa J, and Rabson AS: *Generalized Kaposi's sarcoma is not a neoplasm. Lancet 1: 58, 1983.*

Wuerthele-Caspe Livingston V: *Cancer: A new Breakthrough. Nash Publishing, Los Angeles, 1972.*

Moss RW: *Livingston and the cancer microbe. In, The Cancer Syndrome, Grove Press Inc., New York, 1980, pp 199-211.*

Cantwell AR Jr: *Variably acid-fast bacteria in vivo in a case of reactive lymph node hyperplasia occurring in a young male homosexual. Growth 46: 331-336, 1982.*

Netterberg RE, and Taylor RT: *The Cancer Conspiracy, Pinnacle Books, New York, 1981.*

15 Mycobacteria in AIDS

"We wish to alert physicians who examine bone marrow biopsies from patients with AIDS about the possibility of occult marrow infection by Mycobacterium avium-intracellulare. We have recently cared for two patients in whom infection by atypical mycobacteria was unsuspected. Since our initial experience with these two cases, five more patients with AIDS have had identical biopsy findings. We would recommend that acid-fast staining be done routinely whenever a bone marrow biopsy is performed on any patient with AIDS, Kaposi's sarcoma, or hairy cell leukemia." Cohen RJ, *et al*: Occult infection with M. intracellulare in bone marrow biopsy specimens from patients with AIDS. The New England Journal of Medicine 308:1475-1476, June 16, 1983.

It is difficult to imagine doctors treating patients one hundred years ago. Doctors knew nothing about bacteria and viruses. There was no such thing as the immune system. Antibiotics did not exist. Although one or two microscopes might exist at a medical school, most doctors had never peered inside one. The microscope was still considered a curious instrument, but hardly useful for medical diagnosis. Without knowledge of microbes, and infectious diseases, medicine in the nineteenth century was little more than a science founded on folk medicine, folklore, and superstition.

The first person to ever see a microbe was neither a doctor, nor a scientist, but a curious Dutchman named Antony van Leeuwenhoek, who was born over 350 years ago, and who worked as a draper in the city hall in Delft. His occupation would hardly have led to his eventual fame, were it not for his life-long obsession for grinding glass lenses. He ground the most beautiful and powerful lenses anyone had ever seen. By mounting these lenses, he fashioned the first microscope which could magnify objects, up to three hundred times. Leeuwenhoek spent his life studying, recording, and illustrating many forms of microscopic life.

Leeuwenhoek dutifully shared his microscopic findings with the Royal Society of England, a scientific society which took great interest in the "tiny animals" that could be seen wiggling and swimming under the powerful hand-made lenses which he had so carefully ground. Leeuwenhoek died in 1723, at the age of 91. Strangely, it would be another century and a half until someone realized that these microscopic "animacules" were the cause of infectious diseases, which would continue to plague mankind up to the present time.

The father of modern medicine was not a doctor, but the great French chemist, Louis Pasteur (1822-1895). During the 1860s, Pasteur's experiments proved, beyond doubt, that bacteria and other microbes were the cause of fermentation, decay, and decomposition. Pasteur eventually became world-renowned for his development and use of the rabies vaccine. Before the Pasteur vaccine treatment of rabies, this viral disease was always fatal, and people bitten by rabid animals suffered horrible deaths.

During the closing years of the nineteenth century, Pasteur shared world fame with his scientific rival, Robert Koch (1843-1910). Koch was a German country doctor, twenty one years younger than Pasteur. In 1871, at age 28, his wife presented him with his first microscope. Koch quickly became fascinated with his microscopic studies, and obsessed with the idea that microbes were somehow involved in producing human and animal diseases. The first disease that Koch studied was anthrax, an epidemic disease of cattle, and an uncommon but dreaded disease of man.

Koch learned how to grow bacteria in the laboratory, first on potato skins, and later, in "pure culture" on gelatin mixtures. He injected anthrax microbes into mice and observed their lethal effects. In 1876, after five years of study, he presented his microscope, his mice, his bacteria, and his experimental findings, to the scientific faculty at the University of Breslau. At age 34, Koch convinced the doctors that bacteria were the cause of anthrax.

Koch became the most famous doctor the world had ever known. In 1882, he announced his most important discovery. He declared that tuberculosis, the most feared disease of that time, was caused by a bacterium. Koch had observed the microbe, the "tubercle bacillus," in all cases of tuberculosis he had studied. He was able to grow the bacterium in pure culture. The bacillus could be stained and observed microscopically. Mice injected with the "TB" germs quickly died, and the tubercle bacilli could be regrown in culture from the diseased tissue of the mice.

Koch claimed that in order to prove, beyond doubt, a microbe caused a particular disease, it was first necessary to produce the disease in healthy animals, by infecting them with pure cultures of the microbe. The animals must then succumb to a similar disease, and the germ must be able to be regrown from the diseased animal's affected tissue. These necessary scientific procedures for proof of infectious disease, became known as "Koch's postulates."

Koch's discovery of the tubercle bacillus, later named *Mycobacterium tuberculosis*, revolutionized medical thinking. Previously, tuberculosis was regarded as a hereditary disease, often brought about by poor diet.

A few years later, *Mycobacterium avium* was found to be the cause of fowl and swine tuberculosis, and *Mycobacterium bovis* the cause of TB in cattle.

In 1874, eight years before the discovery of the

mycobacterium of tuberculosis, Gerhard Hansen, a Norwegian physician, had discovered, (in the diseased tissue), the mycobacterium that causes leprosy. The microbe was later named *Mycobacterium leprae*, and leprosy is now known as "Hansen's disease." Although microbes have been grown from leprosy tissue, these microbes are not "accepted" as the leprosy mycobacterium. Most scientists claim that the leprosy microbe cannot be grown outside the human body. Although Koch's postulates have never been proven in Hansen's disease, all scientists agree that leprosy is a mycobacterial infection.

There are many different kinds, or "species," of mycobacteria which abound in the environment, including one species, (*Mycobacterium smegmatis*), which may be found in smegma, the cheesy glandular secretions of the foreskin of the penis. Mycobacteria, other than those causing tuberculosis and leprosy, were never thought to cause human disease. But by the 1950s, medical scientific opinion was again proven wrong. It was becoming increasingly clear that some "atypical," harmless, and "saprophytic" mycobacteria were causing serious, and sometimes fatal disease, in human beings.

All species of mycobacteria have one feature in common. All mycobacteria are "acid-fast" when stained with certain dyes, such as carbol fuchsin. In order to search for acid-fast mycobacteria in diseased tissue, pathologists dye their thinly cut tissue sections with acid-fast stains, such as the Ziehl-Neelsen stain, and the Fite stain. The thinly cut sections are stained *blue* by these methods, and *in contrast*, the mycobacteria are stained red (*acid-fast*).

Mycobacterium intracellulare, an acid-fast mycobacterium that has been found in some AIDS patients, was first discovered in 1949, in a three year-old white girl from North Carolina. She was hospitalized with vomiting, weight loss, anemia, and swollen glands. A tumor, thought to be a cancer (lymphosarcoma), was discovered in her abdomen. The child was given blood transfusions and the tumor was treated with radiation therapy. A lymph gland, removed from her groin, contained acid-fast bacteria. Tissue removed from ulcerated areas of the intestines also showed similar acid-fast microbes.

Despite treatment, the child became emaciated, and died four months after the onset of her illness. At the autopsy, acid-fast bacteria were found inside the cells (intracellular) of the lungs, liver, and spleen. The microbe was isolated in culture, and had the appearance of an acid-fast "fungus," rather than a bacterium. In 1965, microbiologists decided the "fungus" was better classified as a mycobacterium (*Mycobacterium intracellulare*). John Cuttino, a pathologist, and Anne McCabe, a bacteriologist, who reported the original case, noted that if the acid-fast microbes had not been discovered within the tissue, the child would have been considered as having cancer, rather than a fatal bacterial infection.

Since the little girl's death, *Mycobacterium intracellulare* has been found in patients having diseases resembling either tuberculosis, or cancer. But strangely, the mycobacterium can also be isolated from *healthy* people! Cases of this mycobacterial infection have been reported not only from America, but also from South Africa. *Mycobacterium intracellulare* so closely resembles *Mycobacterium avium*, the microbe causing tuberculosis in birds, that microbiologists recently have agreed to join and to classify the two microbes together as *Mycobacterium avium-intracellulare*.

The first reports of *Mycobacterium avium-intracellulare* (MAC) infection in AIDS patients, appeared in 1982. An emaciated, 36 year-old gay man from Houston, Texas, with Kaposi's sarcoma, Pneumocystis pneumonia, and cytomegalovirus infection, also had MAC infection of his lymph glands. Despite anti-tuberculosis medication, he died several months later. At the autopsy, MAC infection was discovered in the lungs, spleen, bone marrow, and in numerous lymph glands.

Phillip Zakowski, *et al* (1982), reported that eight of nine autopsied cases of AIDS at the UCLA Medical Center in Los Angeles, had died with MAC infection, and with "other severe infections." Carl Sohn, *et al* (1983), commented on the similarity between MAC infection and leprosy, in an additional autopsy study of two of these same cases, dying at UCLA.

Five similar cases of AIDS, with four deaths, were reported by Jeffrey Green, *et al*, from the New York City area. The physicians emphasized the rarity of MAC infection, *except* in patients who are immunodepressed. They also commented that "we believe our (five) patients were not normal hosts. Four were homosexual, and one was a drug abuser."

In 1983, a 27 year-old heterosexual man with hemophilia, and Pneumocystis pneumonia, from Ohio, developed fatal MAC infection. The man had been treating himself with "Factor VIII plasma concentrate" for his hemophilia. It was thought the transmissible agent of AIDS might have been acquired through the use of this blood product. One of thirteen AIDS cases from New York City, reported by Catherine Small, *et al* (1983), also died of MAC infection and Pneumocystis pneumonia. The patient was a 24 year-old, heterosexual, Puerto Rican drug abuser.

Scientists are not sure how MAC infection is acquired. According to an editorial by Henry Masur, in *The Journal of the American Medical Association*, (December 10, 1982), "The MAC is present in dust, dirt, fresh water, ocean water, and animal feed. These organisms can be found in birds, including chickens, in the lymphatic tissue of swine, sheep, and cattle, and in eggs, dairy products, and meat. Investigators have found these organisms in 8 to 40% of sputum, tonsil, or urine samples, especially in rural areas. Whether transmission to humans is caused by exposure to inanimate sources and animals, or whether transmission occurs from person to person is unclear."

But MAC mycobacteria are not the only type of mycobacteria affecting high risk AIDS patients. Out of twenty Haitians with AIDS, reported by Arthur Pitchenek, *et al* (1983), from the Miami area, seven had widespread tuberculosis, due to *Mycobacterium tuberculosis*. The TB infection had preceded the development of other infections by 2 to 15 months. Apparently, none of the Haitians were homosexuals, or intravenous drug abusers. Occasional cases of gay men with AIDS have also been found to have tuberculosis, in addition to other opportunistic infections.

Although little known, black Africans with Kaposi's sarcoma often have pre-existing mycobacterial infection with *Mycobacterium leprae*, the bacterium causing leprosy. As cited earlier in Chapter Four, speakers at the 1980 African Symposium on Kaposi's Sarcoma, made clear that leprosy was "astonishingly associated" with Kaposi's sarcoma.

The actual incidence of infection with acid-fast mycobacteria in AIDS patients, is not known. As indicated, infection with acid-fast mycobacteria may be occult.

Are mycobacteria simply "opportunistic agents," or could they possibly *cause* AIDS, at least in some instances? The "connection" between mycobacteria and AIDS is peculiar. Black Africans with Kaposi's sarcoma often have leprosy, due to acid-fast mycobacteria. Black Haitians with AIDS have a high rate of tuberculosis, another common acid-fast mycobacterial infection. Some white, and black American gay men with AIDS have "atypical" tuberculosis due to acid-fast MAC mycobacteria.

The idea of acid-fast mycobacteria as *causative* agents in AIDS might be dismissed, if it were not for several curious findings. Variably acid-fast bacteria have been observed *within the tumors* of both "classic," and "gay" Kaposi's sarcoma. Similar microbes have been found *within the enlarged lymph glands and other organs of AIDS patients.* Equally important has been the century-old finding of acid-fast bacteria in *many different kinds of human and animal cancer*.

Could it be possible that scientists have been overlooking important *bacteriologic* findings in AIDS, by concentrating heavily on the virus theory of AIDS?

A serious error was made in the last major American

116

epidemic when scientists quickly eliminated bacteria as possible causative agents in Legionnaires' disease. What did scientists finally learn about the "tricky" Legionella bacteria which produced occult, and often fatal, lung infections in that famous epidemic? And could a study of the legionnaires' epidemic help us to solve the new epidemic of AIDS?

References

De Kruif P: *Microbe Hunters. Harcourt, Brace and Company, Inc., Cornwall, New York, 1926.*

Cuttino JT, and McCabe AM: *Pure granulomatous nocardiosis: A new fungus disease distinguished by intracellular parasitism. Amer J Pathol 25: 1-47, 1949.*

Jenkin DJM, and Dall G: *Lesions of bone in disseminated infection due to Mycobacterium avium-intracellulare group. J Bone Joint Surg 57-B: 373-375, 1975.*

Fainstein V, Bolivar R, Mavligit G, *et al: Disseminated infection due to Mycobacterium avium-intracellulare in a homosexual man with Kaposi's sarcoma. J Infect Dis 145: 586, 1982.*

Zakowski P, Fligiel S, Berlin GW, *et al: Disseminated Mycobacterium avium-intracellulare infection in homosexual men dying of acquired immunodeficiency. JAMA 248: 2980-2982, 1982.*

Sohn CC, Schroff RW, Kliewer KE, *et al: Disseminated Mycobacterium avium-intracellulare infection in homosexual men with acquired cell mediated immunodeficiency: A histologic and immunologic study of two cases. Amer J Clin Pathol 79: 247-252, 1983.*

Greene JB, Sidhu GS, Lewin S, *et al: Mycobacterium avium-intracellulare: A cause of disseminated life threatening infection in homosexuals and drug abusers. Ann Intern Med 97: 539-546, 1982.*

Elliott JL, Hoppes WL, Platt MS, *et al: The acquired immunodeficiency syndrome and Mycobacterium avium-intracellulare bacteremia in a patient with hemophilia. Ann Intern Med 98: 290-293, 1983.*

Small CB, Klein RS, Friedland GH, *et al: Community acquired opportunistic infections and defective cellular immunity in heterosexual drug abusers and homosexual men. Amer J Med 74: 433-441, 1983.*

Masur H: *Mycobacterium avium-intracellulare: Another scourge for individuals with the acquired immunodeficiency syndrome. JAMA 248: 3013, 1982.*

Pitchenik AE, Fischl MA, Dickinson GM, *et al: Opportunistic infections and Kaposi's sarcoma among Haitians: Evidence of a new acquired immunodeficiency state. Ann Intern Med 98: 277-283, 1983.*

Kaposi's sarcoma: *Discussions of Clinical Features, In Antibiotics Chemother 29: 68-69, Karger, Basel, 1981.*

Cantwell AR Jr: *Bacteriologic investigation and histologic observations of variably acid-fast bacteria in three cases of cutaneous Kaposi's sarcoma. Growth 45: 79-89, 1981.*

Cantwell AR Jr: *Variably acid-fast bacteria in vivo in a case of reactive lymph node hyperplasia occurring in a young male homosexual. Growth 46: 331-336, 1982.*

16 The Lessons of Legionnaires' Disease

Four thousand legionnaires and their families convened at the Bellevue-Stratton Hotel, Philadelphia, in July 1976, for their annual convention. Toward the end of the meeting some conventioners became deathly ill. Their chests and muscles ached. A dry cough began. Chills followed, along with dangerously high fevers, and delirium. Two hundred twenty two people eventually developed the disease, which was quickly termed "legionnaires' disease." Thirty four people died. Pathologists discovered a severe pneumonia-like disease in the lungs of the fatal cases.

Within days, the CDC was notified. An intensive search was undertaken by epidemiologists and medical scientists, to determine the cause of the outbreak. The investigation centered around the hotel, the apparent source of the new epidemic.

For over five months, the cause of legionnaire's disease remained a mystery. Was the disease caused by a poison, a virus, a bacterium, a fungus, or some sort of microbial toxin? Was the disease spread by air, water, food? Could this epidemic be the beginning of "swine flu," which was expected during the winter of 1976.

Despite intensive microbiologic examinations, using the

118

most sophisticated equipment and techniques available, no organism could be isolated from the diseased tissue, nor could any microbe be seen *within* the tissue, either by use of the light microscope, or the powerful electron microscope, which could magnify objects 100,000 times or more.

Extensive laboratory studies were undertaken by scientists at the CDC, in an attempt to transfer the disease to animals. Groups of laboratory animals were inoculated with tissue from victims of legionnaires' disease, but none of the animals became sick, except for the dozen guinea pigs inoculated by Joe McDade.

Joe McDade was a 36 year-old research microbiologist at the Leprosy and Rickettsia Branch of the CDC, which was headed by his superior, Charles Shephard. McDade had inoculated twelve guinea pigs with the diseased lung tissue of three fatal cases of the new epidemic disease. Four of the guinea pigs, inoculated with the tissue of one victim, remained healthy. But six of eight guinea pigs, inoculated with the tissue of two other victims, became ill with fever. When the animals were sacrificed and studied, no microbes could be observed, nor could any microbes be grown from the diseased tissue.

In "Anatomy of an Epidemic" (1982), an historical account of the legionnaires' disease epidemic, Gordon Thomas, and Max Morgan-Witts wrote, "Throughout the CDC other scientists, conducting quite different experiments, were equally unsuccessful in their attempts to isolate the agent. A few, much to Shephard's chagrin, suggested that McDade's guinea pigs became sick as a result of 'some kind of contaminant' or even that 'all guinea pigs get fevers.' Shephard knew animals in his labs didn't normally develop fevers without very good reason: he felt confident they hadn't become ill because of any contamination unwittingly introduced during the tests. Shephard and McDade concluded it was much too soon to give up the search. Perhaps there was something in those guinea pig slides that McDade had so far failed to spot."

McDade never gave up. "On Monday, December 27

(1976), Joe McDade, for reasons that he would remain not exactly clear about, decided to interest himself again in the legionnaires' disease agent. He opened his box containing the slides from two victims. After lengthy microscopic study of the slides, McDade saw what he had not seen in August — the presence of a new bacterium. It was the causative agent of legionnaires' disease."

The discovery of the cause of legionnaires' disease was announced to the world at a press conference held at the CDC, on January 18, 1977. McDade explained the difficulty he had had in detecting the microbe within the diseased tissue. "He and Shephard had decided to rerun their tests with one major change: they would exclude from the embryonated hens' eggs the bacteria-killing antibiotics they had previously used. It made all the difference. The eggs died, fatally infected by the bacteria, which were now able to flourish and reproduce inside them."

The "new" bacterium was named *Legionella pneumophila*. The lessons of legionnaires' disease are that bacteria can still escape detection by expert medical scientists, physicians, pathologists, infectious disease experts, and microbiologists. Bacteria can even be overlooked, or ignored, by virologists looking through powerful electron microscopes. In addition, some kinds of bacteria can refuse to grow in all kinds of routine media for culture, as was the case of the Legionella bacterium. Bacteria which are lethal for humans may cause no disease when injected into laboratory animals.

Physicians, who had unsuccessfully treated fatal cases of legionnaires' disease, were amazed that high-powered antibiotics were not effective in killing Legionella bacteria. Surprisingly, erythromycin, a common and inexpensive antibiotic, is curative in many cases of legionnaires' disease, *if given early* in the disease.

Microbiologists are still astonished that Legionella could not be stained, or detected, in the diseased tissue by use of the "Gram stain," a routine coloring method heretofore successfully used to color all bacteria.

The source of the epidemic in Philadelphia was found to be Legionella bacteria harbored within the air conditioning system of the hotel. The bacteria were apparently scattered into the air by the hotel's cooling system. When inhaled into the lungs of susceptible people, the microbe could cause a fatal pneumonia. The epidemic disease was infectious, but not contagious.

Since the original epidemic, Legionella has been found in the water supply system of some hospitals, resulting in the deaths of some patients. Such hospital-acquired infections are termed "nosocomial" infections.

Although scientists initially thought legionnaires' disease was a "new" disease, and a unique epidemic, we now know that the same microbes were causative of so-called "Pontiac fever," a flu-like, non-pneumonia illness, which broke out in Michigan, in 1968. Another epidemic caused by Legionella bacteria occurred in an engine assembly plant in Windsor, Ontario, in 1981. Within a one-week period, 395 people became ill. The source of the bacteria was an oil-based, contaminated coolant.

Another closely related pneumonia-like disease is caused by a separate species of Legionella, previously called "the Pittsburgh pneumonia agent," and now called *Legionella micdadei* in honor of Joe "McDade." Twenty persons from the Pittsburgh and Virginia areas have been identified as having the pneumonia, since the discovery of *Legionella micdadei*, in 1979. Some of these people were "immunocompromised." Others were normal.

Although the epidemic is officially over, cases of legionnaires' disease continue to occur. Ironically, many reported cases are acquired within hospitals. Victor Yu stated (1982), that more than 100 cases of Legionella infection occurred at the VA Hospital, in Pittsburgh, during a three-year period. Yu contends that these organisms cause unrecognized disease in other hospitals, as well. "You can't find a hospital in the world that doesn't have Legionella in the water supply. In one hospital, that looked at the problem properly, they found that 15% of nosocomial pneumonia was due to Legionella."

In the same report, David Fraser emphasized the possible true incidence of hospital and community-acquired cases of legionnaires' disease, by stating "there is clearly underreporting of legionnaires' disease in the United States. There are probably 25,000 cases per year, but only 200 are reported."

Robert Muder, and a group of physicians, also from the Pittsburgh VA Hospital, undertook a study (1983) to prove that legionnaires' disease also existed at a nearby community hospital. The group reported that "most hospitals have yet to record a case of nosocomial legionnaires' disease; the importance of isolation of *Legionella pneumophila* in the water system of such an institution is unclear. We undertook a prospective pneumonia study in tandem at a veterans' hospital where legionnaires' disease was known to be endemic, and at a community teaching hospital, where legionnaires' disease had never been documented. Legionella serologic tests were performed on all patients with pneumonia; selective culture media and direct flourescent antibody testing for Legionella were made readily available. Simultaneous environmental surveys for Legionella were performed. At the community hospital, we discovered that 64% of sites in the water distribution system yielded *Legionella pneumophila*, and that 14.3% of nosocomial pneumonias were legionnaires' disease."

Originally a "new" disease in 1976, legionnaires' disease is now treatable, although it is still a serious and sometimes fatal illness. Initially, the true bacterial cause of the epidemic was not recognized because all tests were "negative" for bacteria. But what if a special microscopic stain, or a special culture medium, was necessary to uncover a bacteriologic agent in the "new" epidemic of AIDS. Can we be sure the experts are correct by focusing their attention on a new viral agent?

In "Anatomy of an Epidemic," the authors wrote "in the laboratories of the Viral Pathology Branch, scientists conducting electron microscopic studies of legionnaires' lung tissue were so far seeing only what they expected to see: the sort of bacteria that pile up in the lungs of people who die of pneumonia."

Medical scientists have often overlooked, ignored, or have failed to recognize, pathogenic bacteria, (and other microbes), in previous epidemics. It is often said, "history repeats itself." After we review the century-old existence of the "cancer microbe," we will provide evidence to suggest that bacteria are again being disregarded as causative agents in the current AIDS epidemic.

References

Strausbaugh LJ: *Legionnaires' disease. Intl J Dermatol 22: 239-244, 1983.*

Thomas G, and Morgan-Witts M: *Anatomy of an Epidemic. Doubleday & Company, Inc., Garden City, New York, 1982.*

Knudsen F, Nielsen AH, Hansen KB, *et al: Legionella micdadei (Pittsburgh pneumonia agent) may cause nonpneumonic legionellosis. Lancet 1: 708, 1983.*

Isenberg HD: *Microbiology of legionnaires' disease bacterium. Ann Intern Med 90: 502-505, 1979.*

Medical News: *Sometimes getting into hot water solves a (Legionella) problem. JAMA 248: 2793-2795, 1982.*

Muder RR, Yu VL, McClure JK, *et al: Nosocomial legionnaires' disease uncovered in a prospective pneumonia study. JAMA 249: 3184-3188, 1983.*

17   The Cancer Microbe

It was only the recognition of disease-producing bacteria in the nineteenth century, that allowed medical science to emerge from the dark ages, into the era of "modern" medicine. Unfortunately, medical science in the twentieth century has failed in one important aspect. Both the cause and cure of human cancer remain unknown and elusive.

For a physician, (or any individual), to suggest that cancer is caused by bacteria, which can be seen easily in an ordinary microscope, would appear to be an outrageous pronouncement. Most medical scientists have always considered the idea of a bacterial "cancer microbe" as preposterous.

In general, doctors remain firmly convinced that bacteria are not associated with cancer because this is what they were taught in medical school. Nevertheless, we will now briefly discuss the century-old existence of the cancer microbe, and the evidence for its role as the causative infectious agent of cancer.

Cancer is an infectious disease caused by variably "acid-fast" bacteria. The cancer microbe exists in the blood and tissues of all human beings and animals. It is found in people who are healthy, as well as in people who are sick. The organism is "pleomorphic," which means it may appear in many different forms. These forms range in size from submicroscopic forms resembling viruses, up to the size of much larger forms resembling yeasts, fungi, and parasites.

The shape of a bacterium is governed by its cell "wall," much like the shape of a human being is governed by the bones of the skeletal system. Bacteria are highly adaptive. In order to survive and exist within the human body, a bacterium may shed its cell wall. Such bacteria are then known as "cell wall deficient bacteria."

The cancer microbe is cell wall deficient. By shedding its "wall," the cancer microbe may escape destruction by the body's immune system. When the body's immune system becomes unbalanced, (for whatever reason), these cell wall deficient cancer microbes may become pathogenic, and produce cancer, and other diseases.

Bacteria were dismissed as the cause of cancer in the beginning of this century. The reasons were clear. Cancer was proclaimed to be both a non-infectious and noncontagious disease. "Microbes," originally observed in microscopic sections of cancer tissue, were later re-interpreted as cell degeneration, or merely as unimportant bacterial invaders of tissue weakened by cancer. All microbes, grown *in the laboratory* from cancer tissue, were likewise thought to be either "secondary bacterial invaders," or bacterial "contaminants" of laboratory origin.

In the light of all this authoritative scientific opinion, researchers who continued to be interested in the bacteriology of cancer were assumed to be persons of unsound and unscientific mind.

In 1890, William Russell (1852-1940) was the first to see microbes in cancer tissue, which he termed "cancer parasites." Russell, a pathologist from Edinburgh, Scotland, used special tissue staining methods to detect cancer parasites, which he found both within the cells (intracellular) and outside of the cancer cells (extracellular). Some parasites were so tiny Russell could barely observe them in his tissue preparations. Other forms were very large, approximating, and even exceeding, the size of red blood cells. Microbes were found in almost every cancer tumor Russell examined. But *similar* parasites could also be found in tuberculosis and other diseases.

Russell's parasites are well-known to pathologists, but the so-called parasites are now called "Russell bodies," of nonmicrobial origin. For many years, Russell bodies have been assumed to be "immunoglobulins" produced within "plasma cells." However, a recent immunologic and electron microscopic study by Su-Ming Hsu, *et al*, has challenged this traditional belief. Although Russell bodies were discovered almost a century ago, Hsu maintains their precise origin and nature still remain unknown.

Before the close of the nineteenth century, a variety of microbes had been cultured from cancer tissue. They were described as "cancer coccidia," "blastomycetes," "sporozoons," and "amoeboid parasites." Some microbes had the appearance of "Russell bodies." A few organisms even produced cancer tumors when injected into laboratory animals. But the varied microbes cultured from cancer, (many of which probably were laboratory contaminants), combined with the inability of microbiologists to consistently produce experimental cancer tumors in animals, with these so-called cancer microbes, finally led to the general abandonment of the parasitic theory of cancer.

By the 1920s, only a handful of people were using the young science of bacteriology to unmask the secrets of microbes isolated from cancer. In 1921, James Young, an obstetrician from Scotland, reported his findings of a cancer organism which had a "specific life cycle." The "youngest stage is minute, being just recognizable under the highest power of the microscope." These tiny microbial forms were described as "spore forms," and Young was successful in growing them in his laboratory. The "spores" rapidly transformed into larger "coccoid" (round) forms, and rod-shaped bacillary forms. All these microbial forms continued to enlarge into large "spore balls." These spores balls could be seen within the cancerous tissue.

Young, in 1925, claimed the cancer parasite belonged to familiar bacteria, which were ubiquitous in nature. Young injected laboratory animals with these microbes. Not all animals were susceptible to the pathogenic effects of these bacteria. Young stressed that cell susceptibility was the all-important factor in experimentally induced infection with the cancer microbe.

Young's cancer microbe met with a hostile reception. Archibald Leitch, a fellow obstetrician in charge of reproducing Young's experimental cancer studies, was unable to confirm Young's findings. This led to a heated exchange of letters, immortalized in *The British Medical Journal*. Leitch wrote, "I do not grumble at Dr. Young's poor opinion of me, nor at his controversial methods, but I am genuinely sorry that a man of his abilities should waste his time on his so-called ' cancer parasites ' — what my old teacher, Professor George Buchanan, would have described as just a wee lump of *dirt*."

During the 1920s, the idea of a cancer parasite was kept alive in America, by John Nuzum, a Chicago physician. Nuzum studied a pleomorphic "coccus" which he grew from breast cancer in mice. He later isolated similar microbes from human breast cancer. These cocci were identical to the "spore forms," described by Young. Some cocci were so minute that they easily passed through a laboratory microbiologic filter designed to hold back bacteria. This indicated that some forms of the cancer microbe were submicroscopic and virus-sized.

Nuzum could not produce experimental cancer in mice. However, breast tumors developed in two of ten female dogs injected repeatedly with the cocci. Nuzum also performed a daring and dangerous experiment in a hospitalized 70-year old farmer. He injected an area of the man's groin with 62 inoculations of his "coccus," which had been isolated from human breast cancer. After 18 weeks, a skin cancer formed in the area. This experiment, a half-century ago, suggested that bacteria isolated from one kind of cancer, such as breast cancer, might be capable of producing another "different" kind of cancer, such as skin cancer.

In 1925, *Northwest Medicine* published two papers by Michael Scott, a Butte, Montana surgeon who became obsessed with the "parasite of cancer," after he had learned of the microbe from T.J. Glover, in 1921. Scott's description of the microbe was similar to Young's. The parasite had a life cycle composed of three stages, a bacillus or rod-like stage, a round coccus-like stage, and a "spore sac" stage. Like Russell, and Young, Scott claimed these cancer parasites could be seen in cancer tissue. Scott also claimed that the microbe produced a "toxin" which induced the cell proliferation and multiplication, in cancer.

Scott likened cancer to tuberculosis. He wrote: "Because tuberculosis was looked upon by physicians and laymen as being non-infectious and non-contagious, proper precautions were not taken to prevent its spread. The result was the awful increase of the disease to the stage where all civilized mankind became appalled at the rapidly growing armies of its victims." "We are positive, that as soon as the medical profession and laity become convinced of the infectious nature of carcinoma (cancer) and its contagiosity, the adoption of preventive measures, which will follow, will effect a lowering of the rate of incidence of this disease, comparable with what obtains today with tuberculosis." Scott was convinced, on the basis of his animal inoculation studies, that immunization against the cancer parasite was possible.

By 1929, a few microbiologists were becoming interested in the possible existence of a cancer microbe. The Stearns, and B.F. Sturdivant, laboratory workers in Pasadena, California, consistently isolated bacteria from malignant tumors. These pleomorphic microbes were impossible to classify bacteriologically. The research microbiologists described and illustrated two complex growth phases of the microbe. The first phase consisted of a "minute coccobacillus, a slightly pointed rod, and a coccus." The second phase consisted of long curved rods, branching forms, minute cocci, and larger cocci. All these growth forms were interrelated. The coccus form of the cancer microbe could not be distinguished from ordinary staphylococcus cultures. But unlike common staphylococci which always retained their round form, the cancer cocci behaved strangely, when grown in the laboratory. Depending on the culture media, the cocci could be made to change into much smaller cocci, and into rod-shaped bacillary microbes!

One year later (1930), Glover was the first to consistently isolate the cancer microbe from the *blood* of cancer patients. He confirmed that the microbe was "filtrable." But he also made new observations. "Old" laboratory cultures of the cancer organism, which were allowed to dry for months, became transformed from "spore bearing bacilli" into fungus-like microbes, with large "spore sacs."

In 1934, Wilhelm von Brehmer, a German physician from Berlin, was the first to describe and illustrate bacteria *within* the blood cells of cancer patients.

Georges Mazet, a French physician, found pleomorphic "acid-fast" bacteria in Hodgkin's disease in 1941, and later reported similar acid-fast bacteria in many different kinds of cancer, including leukemia.

The most daring concepts of cancer were developed by Wilhelm Reich (1897-1957), a highly controversial Austrian physician, who began his studies of cancer in the 1930s in Europe. He continued to advance his cancer theories, as an emigrant to America in the 1940s. Reich defined cancer, not as a tumor, (the tumor being a late manifestation of the disease), but as a "systemic disease," a disease of the whole body. Reich spent his life developing the theory and use of "orgone energy" — a specific life-energy he claimed existed in the atmosphere, and in all living things.

Reich believed bacterial microbes, which he called

"T bacilli," were present in the blood and excreta of all human beings. These microbes were specifically connected with the development of cancer tumors. He wrote that "every cancer patient and every cancer tissue contains masses of T bacilli." According to Reich, the origin of these bacteria was from degeneration of body protein.

Reich grew T bacilli from both healthy and diseased individuals. The microbes grew slowly from healthy people, but grew *quickly and easily* from the blood of cancer patients. Mice, injected with these bacilli, died within 24 hours!

After months of experimentation, Reich concluded that "the distinction between the healthy individual and the cancer patient does not lie in the *absence* of T bacilli, but in the orgonotic potency of the organism, i.e., in the capacity of the organism to *eliminate* its T bacilli, and in the degree to which the tissues, and the blood cells, tend towards disintegration into T bacilli. The disposition to cancer is therefore determined by the biologic resistance of the blood and tissues to putrefaction."

Even more heretical than the proposed role of T bacilli in cancer, was Reich's appraisal of "amoeboid parasites," which he also observed microscopically in cancer tissue. Reich believed these parasites *actually developed from liquifying cancer tissue!*

Reich realized that "the assertion that there is an endogenous infection, or even an organization of protozoa, in the body, sounds *absurd* to every mechanistic pathologist. He will not even listen to such a thing."

To this day, Reich's ideas seem peculiar. However, in view of the multitudinous infectious agents including viruses, bacteria, protozoa, yeasts, and fungi, in AIDS patients with and without cancer, some consideration should be given to Reich's unorthodox views regarding the existence of T bacilli, and amoeboid parasites, in malignancy.

Reich's discovery of orgone energy, and his later development and use of "orgone energy accumulators" as healing instruments, eventually caused the United States Food and

Drug Administration to take legal action against him. Reich was served with an injunction in 1954, and later accused of violating the court order. He was charged with criminal contempt, found guilty, and sentenced to two years in prison. On November 3, 1957, he was found dead in his cell at the Federal Penitentiary in Lewisburg, Pennsylvania.

For almost 40 years, the leading proponent of the bacterial cause of cancer has been Virginia Livingston, a physician from San Diego, California. Livingston, not only showed the cancer microbe both within (*in vivo*) and outside of the human body (*in vitro*), but also described the appearance of the microbe within the blood of cancer patients, by use of the "dark-field" microscope. By means of electron microscopy, she and her co-workers, were the first to photograph the submicroscopic, "filtrable" virus-like forms of the microbe.

Livingston showed the cancer microbe could be identified both *in vivo* and *in vitro*, by its "acid-fast" staining quality. The "red-stained" (acid-fast) appearance of the cancer microbe indicates that this microbe might be related to other acid-fast bacteria, such as the mycobacteria that cause tuberculosis and leprosy.

Livingston was the first to demonstrate that cancer microbes could secrete a "growth" hormone, similar to human choriogonadotropic hormone (HCG). HCG is a hormone secreted by the placenta, the tissue which protects the fetus from destruction by the mother's immune system. Livingston proposes that the secretion of this hormone by the cancer microbe, protects both the microbe *and* the cancer cells, from destruction by the immune system.

Livingston's achievements in cancer microbiology can be found in her autobiographical book "Cancer, a New

Breakthrough" (1972), and in "The Microbiology of Cancer" (1977), and "The Conquest of Cancer" (1984). Many of Livingston's findings have been confirmed by such scientific investigators as Eleanor Alexander-Jackson, Irene Diller, Florence Seibert, Alan Cantwell, Hernan Acevedo, and others.

Bacteriologists have had great difficulty accepting the idea of "pleomorphic" microbes, and question the existence of the many different growth-forms claimed for the so-called cancer microbe. Most microbiologists believe a coccus always remains a coccus. The idea of a bacterium changing from a coccus to a rod, or to a fungus, or to virus-size forms, is completely unacceptable.

According to Livingston, the cancer microbe is a specific, and highly adaptable microbe, which she has named *Progenitor cryptocides*. Depending on its environment, the microbe may attain large size, even larger than a red blood cell. Other forms are submicroscopic and virus-sized. In her laboratory, filtered cultures of the cancer microbe, containing no bacteria, have been observed to transform back into bacterial-sized microbes.

The cancer microbe has adapted to life within man and animals, by existing in a cell wall deficient state. In cancer tissue, the microbe can be seen microscopically as a variably acid-fast (blue, red, or purple-stained) "coccus" or "granule." These forms can be observed both intra- and extracellularly. Occasionally, large, round forms of cancer bacteria resembling Russell's "parasites" can be identified. The "filtrable," virus-like forms of the cancer microbe are submicroscopic, and can only be seen by use of the electron microscope.

The cancer microbe, in all its many guises, can be recognized only with a knowledge of the many diverse morphologic and microscopic forms, which have been described for cell wall deficient bacteria. Microbiologists, such as Lida Mattman, and Gerald Domingue, have emphasized the possible role of these long-neglected cell wall bacteria, as pathogenic agents in human diseases.

Despite the century-long history of the cancer microbe, the idea of a cancer bacterium remains unacceptable to modern medical scientists. However, medical history is studded with examples of medical truths which have taken decades, and even centuries, to be understood and accepted as truths. In general, great advances in medical thought have occurred very slowly, especially in the area of infectious disease.

Physicians refused to peer into microscopes for over one century after Antony van Leeuwenhoek designed the first microscope, in which microbes were made visible. The inability of nineteenth-century physicians to recognize the importance of microbes, and their role in human disease, seems inexplicable to scientists of the twentienth century.

With these historic thoughts in mind, it should hardly be surprising that the century-old denial of the cancer microbe by the medical profession would result in the inability of most scientists and physicians to see, or want to see, the "cancer parasite."

Perhaps with the AIDS crisis, scientists will again be stimulated to search for bacteria. We now suggest that the cancer "parasite" *is* the long-sought-after microbe which causes, *not only cancer and Kaposi's sarcoma, but AIDS, as well!*

References

Russell W: *An address on a characteristic organism of cancer. Brit Med J 2: 1356-1360, 1890.*

Hsu SM, Hsu PL, McMillan PN *et al: Russell bodies: A light and electron microscopic immunoperoxidase study. Amer J Clin Pathol 77: 26-31, 1982.*

Boesch M: *The Long Search for the Truth about Cancer, GP Putnam's Sons, New York, 1960.*

Young J: *Description of an organism obtained from carcinomatous growths. Edinburgh Med J (New series) 27: 212-221, 1921.*

Young J: *An address on a new outlook on cancer: Irritation and infection. Brit Med J, Jan 10, 1925, pp 60-64.*

Leitch A: *Dr. Young's cancer parasite. Brit Med J, April 17, 1926, p 721.*

Nuzum JW: *A critical study of an organism associated with a transplantable carcinoma of the white mouse. Surg Gynecol Obstet 33: 167-175, 1921.*

Nuzum JW: *The experimental production of metastasizing carcinoma in the breast of the dog and primary epithelioma in man by repeated inoculation of a micrococcus isolated from human breast cancer. Surg Gynecol Obstet 11: 343-352, 1925.*

Scott MJ: *The parasitic origin of carcinoma. Northwest Med 24: 162-166, 1925.*

Scott MJ: *More about the parasitic origin of malignant epithelial growths. Northwest Med 25: 492-498, 1925.*

Stearn EW, Sturdivant BF, and Stearn AE: *The ontogeny of an organism isolated from malignant tumors. J Bacteriol 18: 227-245, 1929.*

Glover TJ: *The bacteriology of cancer. Canada Lancet Pract 75: 92-111, 1930.*

Von **Brehmer W:** *"Siphonospora polymorpha" n. sp., neuer Mikrooganismus des Blutes und seine Beziehung zur Tumorgenese. Med Welt 8: 1179-1185, 1934.*

Mazet G: *Etude bacteriologique sur la malade d'Hodgkin. Montpellier Med 1941: 316-328, 1941.*

Mazet G: *Corynebacterium, tubercle bacillus, and cancer. Growth 38: 61-74, 1974.*

Reich W: *The Cancer Biopathy. Ferrar, Straus and Giroux, New York, 1973.*

Wuerthele Caspe (Livingston) V, Alexander-Jackson E, Anderson JA, et al: *Cultural properties and pathogenicity of certain microorganisms obtained from various proliferative and neoplastic diseases. Amer J Med Sci 220: 628-646, 1950.*

Wuerthele Caspe Livingston V, Livingston AM: *Demonstration of Progenitor cryptocides in the blood of patients with collagen and neoplastic diseases. Trans NY Acad Sci 34(5): 433-453, 1972.*

Wuerthele Caspe Livingston V, Livingston AM: *Some cultural, immunological, and biochemical properties of Progenitor cryptocides. Trans NY Acad Sci 36(6): 569-582, 1974.*

Wuerthele Caspe Livingston V: *Cancer, A New Breakthrough. Nash Publishing Corp, Los Angeles, 1972.*

Livingston-Wheeler VWC, Wheeler OW: *The Microbiology of Cancer. Livingston Wheeler Medical Clinic Publication, San Diego, 1977.*

Livingston-Wheeler VWC, Addeo EG: *The Conquest of Cancer. Franklin Watts, New York, 1984.*

Alexander-Jackson E: *A specific type of microorganism isolated from animal and human cancer: Bacteriology of the organism. Growth 18: 37-51, 1954.*

Diller IC: *Growth and morphological variability of pleomorphic, intermittently acid-fast organisms isolated from mouse, rat, and human malignant tissues. Growth 26: 181-209, 1962.*

Seibert FB, Yeomans F, Baker JA, *et al: Bacteria in tumors. Trans NY Acad Sci 34(6): 504-533, 1972.*

Acevedo HF, Slifkin M, Pouchet GR, *et al: Immunohistochemical localization of a choriogonadotropin-like protein in bacteria isolated from cancer patients. Cancer 41: 1217-1229, 1978.*

Cantwell AR Jr, Kelso DW: *Microbial findings in cancers of the breast and in their metastases to the skin. J Dermatol Surg Oncol 7: 483-491, 1981.*

Cantwell AR Jr: *Histologic observations of variably acid-fast coccoid forms suggestive of cell wall deficient bacteria in Hodgkin's disease. A report of four cases. Growth 45: 168-187, 1981.*

Mattman LH: *Cell Wall Deficient Forms, CRC Press, Cleveland, Ohio, 1974.*

Domingue GJ (Ed): *Cell Wall Deficient Bacteria. Basic Principles and Clinical Significance. Addison Wesley Publishing Company, Reading, Mass, 1982.*

18   The Cancer Microbe in Kaposi's Sarcoma

Martin was a 72 year-old Jewish man. In 1971, a growth was removed from his mouth, at a Los Angeles hospital. The pathologist, microscopically examining the red tumor, saw the vascular slits filled with red blood cells, and the cancerous "spindle cells," so characteristic of Kaposi's sarcoma. In April 1972, three more red tumors were excised from Martin's tongue. Six months later, debilitating and unremitting fevers began.

He was hospitalized. Two different bacteria, (*Klebsiella* and *Escherichia coli*), were grown from his blood. The blood infection was eradicated with antibiotics, and chemotherapy for Kaposi's sarcoma was begun.

Within one year, numerous skin tumors of Kaposi's sarcoma had appeared on his arms and legs. His legs became pitifully swollen. He had great difficulty swallowing. Martin was again hospitalized in October 1973, and died within six days. Jerry Lawson, the pathologist, found internal Kaposi's sarcoma tumors of the heart, lungs, intestines, lymph nodes, kidneys, and spleen. He also noted bacteria within the lungs. This finding was peculiar. Martin had shown no signs of infection in the weeks before his death.

Seven years after Martin's death, Alan Cantwell, a dermatologist, decided to look for "cancer microbes" in Kaposi's sarcoma. He reasoned, if bacteria were causing cancer, the microbes should certainly be visible in the autopsy tissue. It was easy to restudy Martin's case. The organ tissue had been "fixed," and embedded into blocks of paraffin. The tissue blocks were retrieved from storage, and thinly recut sections were stained with the acid-fast stain, in order to search for cancer microbes.

No scientific researcher had specifically looked for bacteria in Kaposi's sarcoma, for decades. In 1939, two pathologists, Roger Choisser and Elizabeth Ramsey, had searched for acid-fast, and other kinds of bacteria, in two autopsied cases of Kaposi's sarcoma. No bacteria were found. The pathologists declared that "no etiological agent has ever been demonstrated, (in Kaposi's sarcoma), despite extensive bacteriologic work."

But Cantwell wasn't looking for brightly red-staining, rod-shaped, acid-fast mycobacteria such as the kind one would expect to find in tuberculosis, or leprosy. The cancer microbe was not usually seen in that form. The dermatologist was hunting for "coccoid" and "pleomorphic" forms, which could be stained a pale-red, purple, or blue color, by use of acid-fast stains.

Cantwell found exactly what he was looking for. Variably acid-fast, pleomorphic, coccoid, and rod-shaped bacterial forms were found in the lungs, as previously noted by Lawson. Numerous coccoid forms were seen in the heart, in the Kaposi's sarcoma tumors of the intestines, in the skin tumors of Kaposi's sarcoma, and throughout the connective tissue.

The microbes were present inside and outside of the cancer cells, and were similar to cancer microbes described by other scientists, over the past century. This study, along with photomicrographs of the microbe, was published in 1981, the same year the AIDS epidemic began.

At the same time he was studying fatal Kaposi's sarcoma, Cantwell was also testing skin tumors of Kaposi's sarcoma for bacteria. His patients were three older Jewish men, *who were otherwise well.*

One patient had had Kaposi's sarcoma for over 25 years! After scrubbing the skin with alcohol, a piece of tumor was "punched out" with a biopsy instrument. One part of the skin biopsy specimen was sent to the pathologist for study and diagnosis. The other portion was sent to the bacteriologist to see if bacteria could be grown from the tumor tissue.

Acid-fast coccoid forms were seen within the microscopic sections of the Kaposi's sarcoma tumors in two of the three cases. Bacteria were grown from the Kaposi's sarcoma tumors of two of these men. In one case, corynebacteria and *Propionibacterium acnes* were isolated. In another case, both *Staphylococcus epidermidis* and *Streptococcus viridans* were cultured.

This study, also published in 1981, indicated that bacteria could be grown from Kaposi's sarcoma tumors. Unfortunately, the kind of bacteria that were grown are frequently encountered in bacteriology laboratories, and are often thought of as bacterial "contaminants" of the skin, or as "secondary invaders" of diseased tissue. No one had yet described such commonplace microbes as "opportunistic."

The *microscopic* appearance of Kaposi's sarcoma in gay men with AIDS is indistinguishable from "classic" Kaposi's sarcoma as seen in older, heterosexual men. Cantwell decided to hunt for acid-fast bacteria in AIDS cases with Kaposi's sarcoma.

The microscopic findings of intracellular and extracellular, variably acid-fast coccoid forms, within the skin tumors of two young homosexual men with AIDS, were reported by Cantwell, in July 1983. The bacteria observed *in vivo* within the gay men's Kaposi's sarcoma tumors, were identical to the bacteria observed within the tumors of the older, heterosexual Jewish men.

In Cantwell's 1983 paper, case one was a 31 year-old gay man with fatal AIDS. The man had been previously reported as "patient 3," by Michael Gottlieb, *et al* (December 1981); and as "case 4," by Philip Zakowski, *et al* (December 1982).

This man was first hospitalized in January 1981, at UCLA, in Los Angeles. He'd had a chronic, Candida yeast infection of the mouth for ten years. Tests showed stomach ulcers, and erosions of the esophagus due to Candida. A biopsy of the esophagus showed cell inclusions, characteristic of cytomegalovirus infection.

Special blood tests showed severe immunodeficiency. While hospitalized, he acquired parasitic Pneumocystis pneumonia. Despite medication, both the yeast, and the parasitic infection, could not be controlled. This part of his case study was reported by Gottlieb, *et al*, from UCLA.

Additional details of his case were supplied by Zakowski, *et al*, also from UCLA. External and internal Kaposi's sarcoma tumors appeared two months before his death, in November 1981. A large, foul-smelling abscess developed at an injection site over the left hip. A variety of different bacteria were cultured from this abscess.

Autopsy examination showed cytomegalovirus inclusions of the esophagus, the colon, and the brain. Adenovirus "32" was cultured from the lung tissue, but cytomegalovirus could not be isolated. The lungs were free of Pneumocystis parasites. Tumors of Kaposi's sarcoma were discovered in the lungs, stomach, intestines, and rectum. Bacteria were not identified at the autopsy. The actual cause of death was not clear.

But at the time of the final autopsy report, the results of certain slow-growing mycobacterial cultures taken at the autopsy, had not been received. These autopsy cultures for mycobacteria eventually grew, and were identified as *two* types of "atypical," non-tuberculous mycobacteria (*Mycobacterium avium-intracellulare* and *Mycobacterium gordonae*). A review of acid-fast stained sections of the lungs, spleen, and lymph nodes all showed acid-fast bacteria. Acid-fast bacteria were apparently *not* found within the Kaposi's sarcoma skin tumors, as later reported, in the *same* case, by Cantwell.

The finding of acid-fast mycobacteria in this case of AIDS was reported, *along with seven more AIDS patients* who had died, at UCLA, with similar mycobacterial infections. Only one of nine autopsied cases of AIDS failed to show acid-fast mycobacteria at autopsy.

According to Zakowski, *et al*, acid-fast mycobacterial infection "may have played some role in the death of each of our patients" with AIDS, at UCLA. These mycobacteria are "almost always resistant to conventional anti-mycobacterial therapy and must be treated with four or more drugs." Zakowski's group believed that these mycobacterial infections in their patients occurred late in the course of AIDS, because bacterial cultures taken earlier in the disease, were negative. The mycobacterial infections could have originated "from an old, latent focus of infection, or could have been acquired from the environment" where mycobacteria are common. The UCLA investigators concluded "it was impossible to state whether these atypical mycobacteria had any role in the initial development of the profound cellular defect seen in our patients."

It is impossible to determine if the acid-fast *coccoid* bacteria observed by Cantwell, in the skin tumors of Kaposi's sarcoma occurring two months before the death of this young AIDS patient, had any relationship to the rod-shaped, acid-fast mycobacteria, found at the autopsy, at UCLA. However, both Cantwell, and Zakowki's group were suggesting that acid-fast microbes were playing some role in the cancer tumors, and in the deaths of some gay men, dying of AIDS.

Surprisingly, Kaposi's sarcoma tumors have not been cultured for the possible presence of *ordinary* bacteria. The bacteria cultured from tumors from the two Jewish men studied by Cantwell (1981), were *not* acid-fast mycobacteria. However, these bacteria were identified in Kaposi's sarcoma tumors by using acid-fast staining techniques, which are used to demonstrate acid-fast mycobacteria.

Numerous scientists have observed round, coccoid forms

of bacteria which can develop from the *characteristic rod-shaped form* of mycobacteria. Unless the true (mycobacterial) origin of these aberrant, round, coccoid forms of mycobacteria are known, they simply cannot be identified as mycobacteria. Virginia Livingston, and other scientists, have repeatedly emphasized that *cancer microbes are closely related to mycobacteria.* However, cancer microbes often appear in the diseased tissue, and in culture, as round cocci, *similar in appearance to common staphylococci.*

It is now well-accepted that acid-fast mycobacteria may be one of many opportunistic infectious agents in AIDS. Until the report of T. Scott Croxson, *et al* (1983), in *The New England Journal of Medicine,* no one would have suspected that *typical* mycobacteria could be present *within* the cancerous "spindle cells" of Kaposi's sarcoma tumors in AIDS.

Croxson, *et al,* reported the case of a 43 year-old homosexual man, studied at the Beth Israel Medical Center, in New York City. The patient had enlarged lymph glands, fever, and weight loss. Four months earlier, he had recovered from Pneumocystis pneumonia. *Two* types of mycobacteria were cultured from a lymph node, and a rectal lesion of Kaposi's sarcoma. The two mycobacteria, (*Mycobacterium avium-intracellulare* and *Mycobacterium gordonae*) were the *same two* mycobacteria which were isolated from the previously discussed case of the young man who had died at UCLA.

The doctors at Beth Israel concluded "although atypical mycobacterial infection and Kaposi's sarcoma are both important components in the clinical spectrum of AIDS, the demonstration of atypical mycobacteria, within tissues involved with Kaposi's sarcoma was a surprise to us. Pathologists must now consider the diagnosis of atypical mycobacterial infections, or other types of infections, *in all tissues taken from patients with AIDS.*" (Author's italics)

Three years after the AIDS epidemic began, mycobacteria were still being considered as opportunistic agents. These acid-fast microbes were suspected of "moving in" at the later stages of AIDS, when death was near. But could these mycobacteria be the *cause* of AIDS? Could they cause the *initial* immunosuppression which might then lead to AIDS, and cancer?

By the summer of 1983, there were several reports which were suggesting acid-fast mycobacteria might be "occult" infectious agents in AIDS. Could it be possible that *acid-fast cancer microbes* might be occult infectious agents as well? Or could acid-fast mycobacteria *and* the cancer microbe possibly be the *same* microbe?

References

Choisser RM, and Ramsey EM: *Angioreticuloendothelioma (Kaposi's disease) of the heart. Amer J Pathol 15: 155-177, 1939.*

Cantwell AR Jr, and Lawson JW: *Necroscopic findings of pleomorphic, variably acid-fast bacteria in a fatal case of Kaposi's sarcoma. J Dermatol Surg Oncol 7: 923-930, 1981.*

Cantwell AR Jr: *Bacteriologic investigation and histologic observations of variably acid-fast bacteria in three cases of Kaposi's sarcoma. Growth 45: 79-89, 1981.*

Cantwell AR Jr: *Kaposi's sarcoma and variably acid-fast bacteria in vivo in two homosexual men. Cutis 32: 58-64, 68, 1983.*

Gottlieb MS. Schroff R, Schanker HM, *et al: Pneumocystis carinii pneumonia and mucosal candidiasis in previously healthy homosexual men. New Engl J Med 305: 1425-1431, 1981.*

Zakowski P, Fligiel S, Berlin GW, *et al: Disseminated Mycobactrium avium-intracellulare infection in homosexual men dying of acquired immunodeficiency. JAMA 248: 2980-2982, 1982.*

Csillag A: *The mycococcus form of mycobacteria. J Gen Microbiol 34: 341-352, 1964.*

Wuerthele-Caspe Livingston V: *Cancer, A New Breakthrough. Nash Publishing Corporation, Los Angeles, 1972.*

Croxson TS, Ebanks D, Mildvan D: *Atypical mycobacteria and Kaposi's sarcoma in the same biopsy specimens. New Engl J Med 308: 1476, 1983.*

19   The Cancer Microbe in AIDS

"What enabled McClintock to see further and deeper into the mysteries of genetics than her colleagues? Her answer is simple. Over and over again, she tells us one must have the time to look, the patience to 'hear what the material says to you,' the openness to 'let it come to you.' Above all, one must have 'a feeling for the organism.'" Evelyn Fox Keller, A Feeling for the Organism: The Life and Work of Barbara McClintock (1983).

People who are seriously ill with AIDS *have more than one disease.* One of every three patients has cancer, such as Kaposi's sarcoma, and most patients have more than one kind of opportunistic infection. Therefore, there is no one cause for all the different infectious diseases that currently are included in the AIDS syndrome.

Since the time of Koch, a century ago, physicians have believed each infectious disease is caused by one specific infectious microbe. For example, the syphilis germ causes syphilis; the tuberculosis mycobacterium causes "TB"; and so on. However, in reality, it is well-known that many patients with serious, chronic, life-threatening diseases have always suffered the effects of infection with more than one microbe. Patients with end-stage tuberculosis, cancer, and chronic infectious diseases often die of infections, which physicians have variously termed as "secondary," "opportunistic," "nosocomial," "community-acquired," or "superimposed" infections. Many of these fatal infections, often acquired shortly before death, are caused by common and ordinary microbes which healthy people with "good" immune systems are exposed to constantly.

Scientists are hunting for an infectious agent believed to immunosuppress the immune system prior to the development of AIDS. In theory, this immunosuppressive agent damages the immune system, weakens the body, and allows the possible development of cancer and opportunistic infection.

At present, it is difficult to precisely define AIDS. There are no specific laboratory blood tests for AIDS. Swollen lymph glands, weight loss, fever, and fatigue, often precede the onset of AIDS. But currently there is controversy as to whether these symptoms actually lead to AIDS, because many patients with these symptoms do not develop the syndrome.

If a microbe causes the initial immunosuppression in AIDS, it is reasonable to assume the organism must be present within the body *before* the development of opportunistic infection and cancer. It should also be present in "healthy" people because studies have indicated that some promiscuous but healthy homosexual men are immunodepressed, and therefore at risk for AIDS.

There is little doubt that the agent of AIDS is contagious, at least in some cases. Whether or not *all* adults with AIDS have acquired the disease through *sexual* contact, is not known.

It is my belief AIDS is initially a bacterial infection induced by cell wall deficient bacteria which are present within the blood stream of all human beings. Guido Tedeschi, and other microbiologists at the University of Camerino, in Italy, have discovered "granules" of bacteria living within the red blood cells of both healthy and ill individuals. Some of these bacteria are acid-fast, a feature shared by the cancer microbe. These ordinarily harmless bacteria may become pathogenic when the immune system is weakened.

Bacteria, including acid-fact mycobacteria, have never been seriously considered as *primary* causative agents in AIDS. Scientists simply do not believe that bacteria cause chronic diseases, such as AIDS and cancer.

It is well-known the human body harbors billions of bacteria, and other microbes. For instance, as many as ten million cocci of *Staphylococcus epidermidis* are normally found within one gram of human feces. Bacteriologic studies performed in the early part of this century have shown that many different kinds of bacteria can reside in both "normal" and diseased lymph glands. This should not be surprising because the purpose of lymph glands is to react against invading infectious microbes, including bacteria.

Nevertheless, most physicians still believe the internal organs and blood of healthy, normal persons are "sterile," and contain no potentially infectious bacteria.

Cantwell (1982), reported the finding of variably acid-fast bacteria within the enlarged lymph glands of the neck of a 39 year-old homosexual man with suspected, "early" AIDS. The bacteria were present within the gland, outside of the gland, and in the surrounding connective tissue. The microbes appeared as intracellular and extracellular, tiny, round, coccoid, and granular forms. The bacteria were identical, in appearance, to bacteria which had previously been described and illustrated in many different kinds of cancer, including Kaposi's sarcoma, Hodgkin's disease, and other lymphomas. Two years after this report, the patient is still alive and well, with no evidence of opportunistic infection, or cancer.

Cantwell (1983), reported similar bacteria throughout the tissue of a 48 year-old homosexual man who died of AIDS. The man had been ill for a year, with fever, fatigue, swollen glands, and muscle-wasting. In the months before death, he developed a chronic cough, enlargement of the liver, and kidney failure. Kaposi's sarcoma was discovered in the esophagus, and small bowel, at the autopsy. Cytomegalovirus was isolated from the lung tissue. The bacteria were seen in the heart, liver, lymph nodes, intestines, testes, adrenal glands, bone marrow, and throughout the connective tissue. Numerous Russell bodies were observed in a lymph node, removed three months before death. As previously discussed, Russell (1890) believed these "bodies" were microbes.

By 1983, other physicians were also discovering "occult" infections with acid-fast bacteria in some cases of AIDS. Richard Cohen, *et al*, at the Children's Hospital and Adult Medical Center, in San Francisco, reported a 39 year-old gay man with AIDS, and Kaposi's sarcoma. Prior to chemotherapy, a bone marrow examination was reported as normal. (The bone marrow produces blood cells). Shortly after chemotherapy was started, a blood infection with *Mycobacterium avium-intracellulare*, was discovered. The original bone marrow tissue was restudied, by restaining the marrow with an acid-fast stain. Numerous acid-fast bacterial rods were then revealed in the marrow, by use of this special stain. Despite vigorous treatment with anti-tuberculosis drugs, the patient died within several weeks. Widespread infection, with acid-fast bacteria and cytomegalovirus, was found at the autopsy.

A second patient with AIDS, a gay man, age 37, was also discovered to have an identical, widespread acid-fast bacterial infection, which was treated successfully with anti-tuberculosis medication. Cohen, *et al*, then found five additional patients with AIDS, and occult acid-fast mycobacterial infections in the bone marrow.

The San Francisco doctors concluded, "It now appears that occult infections with this organism, (*Mycobacterium avium-intracellulare*), would not be apparent from the innocent histologic appearance of a bone marrow specimen on standard hematoxylin-eosin staining, and we would recommend that acid-fast staining be done routinely whenever a bone marrow biospy is performed on any patient with AIDS, Kaposi's sarcoma, or hairy-cell leukemia."

It was now clear that acid-fast staining might reveal hidden mycobacteria in AIDS. Strangely, no one was mentioning the cancer microbe which had been reported over the past few decades, as being acid-fast in cancer tissue.

The finding of occult bacteria in the blood, in the blood-forming organs, in the tumors of Kaposi's sarcoma, and throughout the tissues of some patients with fatal AIDS, suggests that:

1) AIDS may be an occult acid-fast bacterial infection.
2) Certain kinds of cancer *and* AIDS may both be produced by the same, or similar, bacterial microbes.
3) Both cancer and AIDS may be infectious diseases.
4) On the basis of epidemiologic data, Kaposi's sarcoma may be one of the most infectious and contagious forms of cancer.
5) The *origin* of the bacteria which cause AIDS, may be either from bacteria already in the body, (endogenous infection), or by bacteria acquired from the external environment, (exogenous infection), or both.
6) Treatment of "early" AIDS should be vigorous. The use of anti-tuberculosis therapy for occult acid-fast mycobacterial infection might be advantageous.
7) A vaccine might be developed against these bacteria.

Undoubtedly, as the AIDS epidemic progresses, new information will appear which will either support, or deny, the possible role of acid-fast bacteria as causative agents in AIDS.

Still, most scientists are searching for new or mutant viruses, as the most likely cause of AIDS. The greatest deterrent to the study of bacteria in the epidemic was the fact that physicians could not conceive of any causative bacteria which could escape detection by modern scientific laboratory methods available in the 1980s.

But perhaps, the denial of bacteria in AIDS was due to the century-old assumption that bacteria could never be implicated in any form of cancer. The idea of a cancer bacterial microbe was still "taboo."

References

Pinching AJ, Jeffries DJ, Donaghy M, et al: Studies of cellular immunity in male homosexuals in London. Lancet 2: 126-130, 1983.

Tedeschi GG, Bondi A, Paparelli M, et al: Electron microscopical evidence of the evolution of corynebacteria-like microbes within human erythrocytes. Experientia 34: 458-460, 1978.

Brumfitt W, and Hamilton-Miller JMT: Coagulase-negative staphylococci. Intl J Dermatol 22: 232-236, 1983.

Cantwell AR Jr: Variably acid-fast bacteria in vivo in a case of reactive lymph node hyperplasia occurring in a young male homosexual. Growth 46: 331-336, 1982.

Cantwell AR Jr: Necroscopic findings of variably acid-fast bacteria in a fatal case of acquired immunodeficiency syndrome and Kaposi's sarcoma. Growth 47: 129-134, 1983.

Cohen RJ, Samoszuk MK, Busch D, et al: Occult infections with M. intracellulare in bone marrow biopsy specimens from patients with AIDS. New Engl J Med 308: 1475-1476, 1983.

20   The Future of the Epidemic

"Despite the repeated statements of health authorities that for the vast majority of Americans there is little or no risk of falling victim to the disease AIDS, many U.S. adults fear the disease is likely to reach epidemic proportions and do not believe an immediate cure will be found." Los Angeles Times, July 7, 1983.

"I'm dealing with my illness the same way I've dealt with everything else in my life. I know that unless the medical profession comes up with something, I'm going to die. But I'm not afraid of death, I've lived a very full life and I don't regret a single thing."
Relaxing in the living room of his Oakland, California, home, Dr. George Riley, MD, a 39 year-old psychiatrist, speaks quietly and softly about the changes in his life since the morning seven months ago when he discovered the purple lesions in his mouth that soon would be diagnosed as Kaposi's sarcoma.
'There have been many moments when I've felt anger and frustration that the medical field, where I've spent my life, isn't able to help me when I need it. That's kind of difficult to accept.'" The agony of AIDS: An MD's battle. American Medical News, August 5, 1983.

By 1984, the national hysteria concerning the AIDS epidemic was mounting. The reasons were understandable. In March 1982, three hundred cases of AIDS had been reported to the Centers for Disease Control. By January 1984, less than two years later, the CDC had recorded more than three thousand cases. By April 1984, almost four thousand cases were reported.

Many people who acquired AIDS had died. Many others were seriously ill. Pitifully, there was no good medical treatment for the disease. Chemotherapy for Kaposi's sarcoma often improved the cancer, but further damaged the immune system, allowing frequently untreatable, and often fatal, opportunistic infections to develop.

Homosexuals, Haitians, hemophiliacs, and heroin addicts, were considered by a sometimes-hostile public, as the most likely spreaders of the disease. To some people, the aberrant lifestyle of people with AIDS, was added proof of the social, moral, and spiritual decline in America.

AIDS is certainly a newly *recognized* disease, but is it really a new disease? A review of the medical literature has suggested that some people have died earlier in this century of AIDS-like illnesses. Other physicians are starting to recall cases of possible AIDS, reported decades ago.

One such case, reported again by George Williams, *et al*, in *The Lancet*, (November 12, 1983), concerned an unmarried Englishman who died in 1959, after a brief illness. Cytomegalovirus and Pneumocystis parasites were found in his lungs at the autopsy. Williams, *et al*, in their report entitled "AIDS in 1959?," remarked that "perhaps AIDS is not a new disease; rare examples may in the past have masqueraded under various guises."

Until a few decades ago, medical science was unaware of the complexity of the immune system. Highly specialized tests to determine the competency of a patient's immune system have only been in wide use for the past two decades. Clinical immunologic blood testing for T and B cell lymphocytes, helper and suppressor cells, monoclonal antibody testing, and other sophisticated tests, have only been in vogue for several years. These immunologic tests are widely used, at present, in the diagnosis of AIDS. But we cannot make the mistake of assuming that AIDS did not exist, before these laboratory tests became available.

It is most probable that cases of AIDS have always been present. The large number of cases, particularly in certain well-defined groups, is undoubtedly a new phenomenon. However, as similar immunologic testing of *all* chronically-ill persons continues, it is entirely possible that many people currently not at risk, will be included in the diagnostic spectrum of AIDS.

The AIDS epidemic has been a disaster for the gay community, and for the medical profession. Health professionals have been powerless to save many patients with AIDS, despite the latest advances in chemotherapeutic drugs, experimental drugs, antibiotics, and top-quality hospital care. When the underlying cause of AIDS becomes known, it will unquestionably contribute to our understanding of both cancer, and opportunistic infection. There is little doubt that AIDS is a pre-cancerous disease, greatly predisposing high risk people, such as gays, to various forms of cancer, particularly Kaposi's sarcoma.

Strangely, AIDS is the only infectious disease in medical history, in which age limits for diagnosis have been established. According to CDC criteria, all persons older than sixty with cancer, are excluded from the diagnosis of AIDS. All patients taking immunosuppressive drugs, and cancer chemotherapy, are also excluded. These already immuno-suppressed groups would appear to be at risk for AIDS, but aged, and cancer patients, have not been studied for AIDS.

All sexually-active male homosexuals are currently at risk. At present, *any* declared homosexual man who is ill, with a poorly-defined disease, will be suspected of having AIDS; particularly, if immunologic tests are abnormal. All gay men are now also considered as potentially abnormal immunologically. Homosexual men are no longer acceptable as blood donors, due to the current belief that the AIDS microbe might be transmitted through blood, and blood products.

My belief, based on research studies, is that AIDS *is* cancer, and that cancer *is* AIDS. The affected tissues of both diseases contain similar-appearing acid-fast bacteria. Although both diseases may be considered "different," the microscopic findings of bacteria strongly suggest that both diseases are due to infection with similar microbes.

Bacteria are found within everyone. They are present in our bodies, even before birth. They probably help us to maintain our health, by keeping other invading microbes in check, and by performing other microbiologic functions, necessary for our survival. But when our immune systems are weakened or damaged, these harmless microbes can become dangerous, and pathogenic.

Although these ideas may seem preposterous to many scientists, these microbes have already been demonstrated in specially-stained microscopic sections of cancer tumors, Kaposi's sarcoma, and throughout the tissues of AIDS patients, studied at autopsies. In all these diseases, the bacteria appear as acid-fast coccoid forms which stain red, blue, or purple. Pleomorphic bacteria, (staphylococcal, streptococcal, and corynebacteria-like microbes), which have been cultured from cancer tumors, and the blood of cancer patients, have been ignored as microbes of no importance. But as we have indicated, there is evidence, which has been provided over the past century by research scientists in many parts of the world, which indicates these acid-fast microbes actually represent the cancer microbe.

Certainly, cancer is not contagious, as are some other infectious diseases. For instance, leprosy is an infectious and contagious disease. However, it is only contagious for *some* people, who live in close contact, for long periods of time, with untreated people who have the disease. Most individuals have a natural immunity to leprosy, or Hansen's disease, as it is now called. Pleomorphic acid-fast bacteria have been cultured from leprosy, but these microbes, similar to those cultured from cancer, have never been accepted as causative agents, by scientific "authorities."

Unfortunately for patients with cancer, medical science

has never paid serious attention to either the cancer microbe, or to the peculiar appearance of bacteria cultured from cancer. Cancer-associated bacteria may be extremely pleomorphic, with a variety of microbial forms, ranging from round cocci to rod-shaped bacilli, similar to the acid-fast mycobacteria found in tuberculosis, leprosy, and other mycobacterial infections.

It is understandable, from a historical point of view, why medical science has failed to grasp the significance and importance of the cancer microbe. Scientists failed to understand the medical importance of *any* microbe, for over one hundred fifty years after bacteria were first observed by Leeuwenhoek. During the twentieth century, cytomegalovirus (considered by many to be *the* cause of AIDS), was overlooked in tissue, for a half-century. Cytomegalovirus was first erroneously interpreted as a "parasite," and later, again misinterpreted as a tissue "degeneration." The parasite, *Pneumocystis carinii*, which causes most AIDS deaths, was overlooked in lung tissue for a half-century, before it was rediscovered. The clinical importance of "atypical" mycobacteria, as a serious cause of human infection, was not appreciated for almost three-quarters of a century. Legionella bacteria went unrecognized, for almost six months, in the epidemic of legionnaires' disease, in 1976, and went undetected for three decades in "mini-epidemics," until the bacteria were retrospectively discovered.

It would not be too surprising if a cancer microbe had been overlooked, or misinterpreted, for a century.

In this book, I have suggested that the origin, and cause, of AIDS are the microbes we carry normally within our bodies. As individuals, we have to deal not only with *our own microbes*, but we must also deal with *other peoples' microbes*, as well as the microbes in our *food*, and in our *environment*.

The microbes we acquire daily must *mix* with the microbes already present within our bodies. Microbiologists know little about the factors which allow different kinds of microbes to exist together, in harmony, within our bodies.

At present, medical scientists simply cannot deal with the disharmony of microbial agents, which ravage patients with AIDS. Scientists have labelled all these microbes as opportunistic agents.

The revolutionary idea that AIDS, and cancer, are similar bacterial diseases caused by the cancer microbe, allows a possible understanding of AIDS, as *only one of many diseases*, to which *all* human beings are susceptible, regardless of racial and cultural characteristics, and their religious and sexual preferences.

Therefore, it becomes understandable why AIDS patients often develop cancer, and why cancer patients often die of opportunistic infection. The production of cancer by the cancer microbe, is also the reason why patients cured of their cancer often develop a recurrent cancer, or another completely different kind of cancer.

One possible reason for the emergence of the new epidemic of AIDS, is that medical scientists may have unwittingly produced more virulent and more contagious cancer bacteria (or cancer viruses), by the widespread use of chemotherapy, antibiotic therapy, and radiation therapy, in the modern treatment of cancer. If cancer *is* an infectious disease, scientists must then ask themselves whether or not treatment methods of cancer, in the late twentieth century, have changed the aggressive nature of the cancer microbe, and allowed it to produce a different kind of disease, such as AIDS.

Before developing AIDS, many patients have had histories of repeated infections with a variety of microbial agents. It is entirely possible the cancer microbe is made more aggressive, not only by *other* invading microbes, but also by chemotherapeutic drugs, prescribed for their eradication. Undoubtedly, the immune system is important in keeping microbes from harming the body. Cancer-producing microbes might become activated, in situations where the immune defenses are weakened, for whatever reason.

Scientists, who have studied the cancer microbe have never believed that orthodox treatment of cancer by use of surgery, radiation, or chemotherapy, has been effective in the elimination of cancer bacteria.

Although doctors realize a healthy immune system is the body's best defense against cancer and AIDS, it is ironic to realize that the treatment of cancer is often chemotherapy, which is injurious to the immune system. But the argument for chemotherapy is strong. Certain statistics have shown that people with cancer live longer with chemotherapy. However, statistics rarely mention the poor quality of life frequently experienced by cancer patients who undergo chemotherapy. Furthermore, statistics are not compiled of cancer patients, dying as a *direct* result of cancer chemotherapy, and radiation.

Tragically, millions of people throughout the world die annually of cancer, despite the best available treatment.

It is apparent that orthodox medicine must develop new and effective treatment for AIDS, and for cancer. It is unlikely that the medical profession will turn to new methods of healing, or to certain effective, but "unorthodox" methods of treatment, unless patients begin to demand it. "Holistic" doctors attempt to meet needs and requests of some patients interested in healing methods, which attempt to treat not only the body, but the mind and spirit, as well.

AIDS is one of the most important diseases of this century. Like other epidemics in the past, it has made mankind realize the continuing difficulty of living in harmony with potentially infectious microbial agents. Although the science of microbiology is one century old, we have still not recognized the existence, nor the importance, of occult bacteria, and viruses, which normally reside within our bodies. Many diseases of unknown cause, are actually produced by these microbes. If medical science is to succeed in this century, attention must now be directed to these so-called harmless microbes, as potential agents of serious disease.

As human beings, we have dealt with microbes from the very beginning of our physical existence. Science has taught us that at the time of our conception we consisted of an egg (ovum), penetrated by a sperm cell. We were so tiny we could only be seen microscopically. At that moment, we were hardly bigger than some microbes, and smaller than some parasites. *But we survived.*

Scientists have been too preoccupied with physical science to pay much attention to the "life force." As we continue to learn about microbes, we will learn about ourselves. Microbes are the smallest of living creatures, just as each of us once was.

Because microbes cannot be eradicated from our bodies, it is unlikely that diseases, such as AIDS, will ever be eradicated. But our serious illnesses always impel us to look inwardly, to find ways to survive. It is this "life force," stronger than any medicine, which encourages us to live, and endure.

The AIDS epidemic has already encouraged many people to improve the quality of their lives and relationships. For some people who have lovers and friends with AIDS, the epidemic has taught them to love and care more deeply.

Patients always expect doctors to have words of wisdom and advice, concerning their illnesses. I am not sure why some gay men and other high risk people acquire AIDS, while others who have similar lifestyles appear to be unaffected. I believe very strongly in bacteria as the medical cause of AIDS, but that does not explain why certain individuals get AIDS, particularly when the AIDS microbe resides within all of us.

I prefer to think patients with AIDS know better than I, the true reasons for their illness. I believe strongly that people will die when they are ready, and, no doctor will keep a patient alive, who has no will to live.

Our culture makes it difficult for us to be chronically ill. We all know it is normal to die, but somehow we consider it *demeaning* to be ill.

My friend, Phil, taught me a lot about AIDS. The last time I saw Phil, he never looked better. I had never seen him more hopeful, or more optimistic. He was 32 years old.

He had AIDS, and Kaposi's sarcoma. He had seen the best doctors in the city. He had been in and out of one of the best medical centers, and he had the best experimental drugs available for AIDS. During his illness, Phil searched his soul as he had never done before. He was looking forward to the future. He had cast out the "devils" in his psyche, which he believed caused him to get ill, in the first place. Two weeks later, he was dead with Pneumocystis pneumonia.

Many people would say it was tragic. I prefer to think Phil left the world because he was ready to leave it. His illness forced him to take the time to explore his deepest feelings, and spiritual beliefs, and to seriously think about himself, and his place in the world. Near the end of life, he began to like himself again, despite fears about the worth of his talents, and his ability and willingness, to give and receive love. He had gone through a private hell. He knew he could make it. And after all, isn't that why we are all here on this planet. To learn about ourselves, and others. Phil certainly influenced my thinking, in ways I am still discovering.

When the mystery of the AIDS epidemic is uncovered for all to see, and we discover the "lessons" the disease has taught us, it is likely medical science, and humanity, will have made a giant step forward.

"Dying is a biological necessity, not only for the individual, but to insure the continued vitality of the species. Dying is a spiritual and psychological necessity, for after a while the exuberant, ever-renewed energies of the spirit can no longer be translated into flesh." Jane Roberts: The Individual and the Nature of Mass Events. A Seth Book (1981).

21   The HTLV-3 Virus Solution

"George W. Riley, MD (page 152), a 39 year-old Oakland, California, psychiatrist with AIDS, died March 27, 1984. Dr. Riley, who discussed his illness in an American Medical News article (Aug. 5, 1983), was a 1971 graduate of Bowman Gray School of Medicine in Winston-Salem, North Carolina. He completed his residency training at George Washington University in Washington, D.C. After two years in the Army, Dr. Riley settled in the San Francisco area.

After being diagnosed with AIDS in early 1983, Dr. Riley retired from practice. In the article, Dr. Riley described himself as a 'generally optimistic person,' expressing hope that medical researchers would discover a cure for the illness in time to help him." MD with AIDS dies at age 39. American Medical News, June 1, 1984.

On April 23, 1984, government scientists proclaimed to the world that the AIDS mystery was solved. A team of medical researchers, headed by Dr. Robert Gallo of the National Cancer Institute, officially announced to the media that they had isolated the "HTLV-3" virus (human T-cell lymphotropic virus) as the *probable* cause of AIDS.

The new AIDS virus, a member of the "human T-cell leukemia virus" family, had been found in the blood samples of 88% of a group of American AIDS patients. The virus specifically attacked "T-cell" lymphocytes. These specialized white blood "T" cells are vital in the body's defense against infectious disease agents. The virus was found in the semen, the saliva, and even the tears of AIDS patients. Later, scientists were surprised to learn that the virus could also attack cells of the central nervous system and spinal cord.

The AIDS virus is now believed to be closely related to the "visna virus," a virus that causes infection of the central nervous system in sheep. HTLV-3 virus is also related to a group of retroviruses associated with certain forms of human cancer. HTLV-1 virus is believed to cause "T-cell" leukemia found in Japan, Africa, and parts of the Caribbean. HTLV-2 virus apparently causes a rare form of "T-cell" leukemia, known as hairy cell leukemia.

The AIDS HTLV-3 virus is an RNA retrovirus. Retroviruses are unusual in that they contain an enzyme (reverse transcriptase) which allows them to reproduce themselves "backward" by transforming RNA into DNA. This remarkable ability to switch genetic material backward from RNA to DNA defied the long-held scientific dictum that genetic transfer could occur only in one direction, namely from DNA to RNA, and never the reverse.

Margaret Heckler, U.S. Secretary of Health and Human Services, immediately announced that the discovery of the AIDS virus by Robert Gallo would allow the development of a vaccine against AIDS, which would be available by 1986. Her prediction quickly proved erroneous. The virus was soon found to mutate rapidly, making the production of a vaccine difficult, if not impossible. A vaccine might be available in 1990 at the earliest. In 1985, Heckler was asked to resign from her post, and was reassigned to a new government position as Ambassador to Ireland.

Gallo's "discovery" of the HTLV-3 virus was soon challenged by Dr. Luc Montagnier of the Pasteur Institute in Paris. Montagnier claimed he had originally discovered and reported on the AIDS virus one year earlier. His research work was highly regarded by French scientists but had been ignored in America. The French virus, isolated from swollen lymph glands of

AIDS patients, was called LAV (lymphadenopathy-associated virus).

For many months scientists could not determine if the French virus and the American virus were the same virus. At present, it is generally accepted that they are closely related, if not identical. The issue of who first discovered the virus is still not settled in scientific circles.

A blood test called the HTLV-3 "ELISA" (enzyme-linked immunosorbant assay) test became available in 1985 which could detect blood which had been exposed to the AIDS virus. This test is now used by all blood banks to screen out contaminated blood, thereby insuring the safety of blood used in transfusions. Not surprisingly, both French and American scientists were separately staking claim to the patent on the new blood test kits. Millions of these kits would be used throughout the world and would be worth millions of dollars to both the scientists and the pharmaceutical companies promoting them.

The HTLV-3 blood test could not determine whether active live virus was present, *but only detected antibodies to the virus.* The presence of these antibodies indicated only that a person had been exposed to the AIDS virus. By itself, a positive blood test did not mean a person had AIDS. In fact, the vast majority of people who tested positive for AIDS virus antibodies were perfectly healthy.

Although the blood test was not considered a diagnostic test for AIDS, there were exceptions to this rule. For example, physicians might use the test as an additional diagnostic test for AIDS in certain patients where the diagnosis was not certain. In 1985, the CDC changed its previous ruling eliminating AIDS as a diagnosis in patients over the age of 60 with Kaposi's sarcoma. From now on, AIDS could be the diagnosis in these patients *if* the HTLV-3 test was positive. If the blood test was negative, patients over age 60 with Kaposi's sarcoma were not reported as AIDS.

Scientists cleverly avoided the issue of what was causing Kaposi's sarcoma in HTLV-3 negative patients. I wondered how a new virus could possibly cause a century-old form of cancer. There was absolutely no direct link between HTLV-3 infection and the development of Kaposi's sarcoma. This fact didn't seem to deter most AIDS experts who insisted that the new virus was the sole cause of AIDS.

Other newly developed immunologic blood tests to detect AIDS virus antibodies indicated there were serious technical problems (as well as ethical problems) connected with the HTLV-3 ELISA blood test. Although some persons had never been exposed to the AIDS virus, they could test "false-positive." Alternatively, some persons proven infected with the virus might test "false-negative," but for some reason the ELISA test could not detect the antibody. Nevertheless, the ELISA test was judged both a "sensitive" and "specific" test for the AIDS virus. In doubtful cases, a confirmatory immunologic blood test called the "Western blot" test could be used to test for the new virus.

The Council on Scientific Affairs of the American Medical Association (AMA) readily admitted "there are uncertainties surrounding the clinical meaning of a positive test and concerning the incidence of true- and false-positive results." Persons with a positive test would be referred to practicing physicians, who would be "expected to determine the significance of a positive test result, offer sagacious medical counseling on a fatal and incurable disease, and do follow-up studies on a disease that has an incubation period of up to five years. The vast majority of physicians have never seen a case of AIDS, and most are unfamiliar with the management of the disease." (JAMA, September 13, 1985).

According to the Council, "high-risk" people who would likely test positive to the new test included "all men who have had sexual contact with another man, intravenous drug abusers, hemophiliacs, and other persons who have had sexual contact with a person who has had an HTLV-3 infection or who is at increased risk of exposure to HTLV-3."

Depending on whether patients were high or low risk, the Council had two different sets of "guidelines" for positive reactors. Gay men and drug abusers would be advised of the risk of infecting others during intercourse. Low risk people would be advised there is "currently insufficient evidence to warrant a broad restriction on sexual relations. Testing the patient's regular sexual partner may provide better or more information to determine if the test result may be a true- or false-positive result."

As I read this AMA report, I was imagining a possible sexual scenario of a low risk person. "I hate to tell you this, but my doctor told me I had a positive blood test for AIDS. He's not sure exactly what it means. He was wondering if you would take the test to see what your test shows. He says I am absolutely healthy, but wants me back in his office in six months to be sure I am OK. Do you feel like making love tonight?"

The Council's report on the state of the art of AIDS blood testing irritated Charles Ortleb, publisher of the *New York Native*, who wrote, (October 14, 1985), "I am as tired of writing about AIDS as you are of reading about it. However, the American Medical Association has just given us another ridiculous set of guidelines, on which I cannot resist comment. The vulgar stupidity of the science the guidelines are based on demands comment." He ended his detailed commentary, "Why doesn't the AMA save everyone a great deal of money and tell us the test stinks? Please stop insulting us with this garbage science. Do we have a test for HTLV-3 antibody or don't we?"

It was unbelievable and tragic that four years after the onset of the epidemic and more than one year after the discovery of the HTLV-3 virus, there was no successful treatment for AIDS. By February 1986, over 17,000 AIDS cases had been reported.

The statistics did not tell the true story. It was estimated that ten times as many people were suffering from milder forms of AIDS known as "pre-AIDS," or more commonly known as "AIDS-related complex" or "ARC" for short. The medical signs and symptoms of these AIDS-related conditions were varied but often included swelling of lymph glands (nodes), night sweats and fevers, loss of appetite and energy, recurring bouts of diarrhea with serious weight loss, peculiar skin rashes and infections, yeast infections of the mouth, and various other complaints.

The long-term survival rate of "pre AIDS" or "ARC" patients was simply not known. Some would die without developing Kaposi's sarcoma and/or Pneumocystis pneumonia, and would never be recorded as AIDS deaths. Most of these patients were gay men who would die of mysterious and obscure causes. Most would be quickly forgotten by physicians who were devoting their energy to save, usually without success, the ever-increasing number of AIDS patients in their practices.

This depressing state of affairs was finally brought home to the American people by the July, 1985 announcement that Rock Hudson was seriously ill with AIDS. On the advice of physicians, the popular actor flew to Paris to undergo experimental treatment with HPA-23 at the Pasteur Institute. The drug was known to reduce the amount of virus in the blood, but was not curative, and often had toxic effects. Film clips of Hudson's final public appearance with Doris Day were widely shown on television. The shocking physical deterioration of the man, especially marked on his previously handsome face, showed the world the horror of a body ravaged with AIDS.

After a short stay in Paris, Rock Hudson returned home to America. Ten weeks later, he was dead. More than the thousands of AIDS deaths which preceded him, Rock Hudson's tragedy instilled upon a mournful public the seriousness of the ever-increasing AIDS epidemic.

Despite years of medical research at the cost of billions of dollars spent on the study of the immune system and suspected cancer viruses, it was now clear there was no magic drug to improve the damaged immune system in AIDS, nor eradicate the HLTV-3 and other viruses which savagely attacked AIDS patients. Newer drugs, such as the widely acclaimed anti-cancer "wonder" drug Interferon, were clearly disappointing in the treatment of AIDS and Kaposi's sarcoma. Other experimental AIDS drugs such as Suramin, previously used for parasitic African sleeping sickness; Ribavirin, used for respiratory and influenza viruses; Phosphonoformate, used against the herpes virus; Ansamycin, used for mycobacterial infections, such as tuberculosis; and numerous other drugs were being tested. Unfortunately, preliminary treatment reports were not encouraging.

The national AIDS hysteria reached its peak in September 1985, when it became known that children with AIDS would be attending public schools. *Time* (September 23, 1985) reported on these "New Untouchables" in this way: "There are 946,000 children attending New York City schools, and only one of them — an unidentified second-grader enrolled at an undisclosed school — is known to suffer from acquired immunodeficiency syndrome, the dread disease known as AIDS. But the parents of children at P.S. 63 in Queens, one of the city's 622 elementary schools, were not taking chances last week. *As the school opened its doors for the fall term, 944 of its 1,100 students stayed home.*"

The increasing AIDS hysteria was greatly fueled by powerful political and religious leaders, especially those who hated and feared gay people. These self-proclaimed AIDS experts called for a quarantine of persons with AIDS, even though scientific evidence showed the disease was not spreadable from person-to-person unless there was sexual activity. A few religious experts believed the new plague was a result of God's wrath against homosexuals. However, the fact that no lesbian had come down with the disease clearly indicated to some AIDS watchers that the wrath of God appeared to be limited to only gay men.

In March 1985, Haitians were removed from the CDC's list of high risk groups for AIDS. At that time, Haitians comprised 3% of the total AIDS cases. The three remaining high risk groups included male homosexuals and bisexuals (74%), intravenous drug abusers (17%), and hemophiliacs (1%). According to the *Physicians Washington Report* (May 1985), the CDC exclusion of Haitians was based on an "increased understanding of how AIDS is spread." But the actual cause of the Haitian susceptibility to AIDS remained unknown, and some CDC officials apparently still considered Haitians at high risk for AIDS. As a result, the CDC did not recommend a change in Public Health Service policy which refused blood donations from Haitians.

The puzzling relationship between AIDS and Kaposi's sarcoma, (the most common form of cancer found in AIDS), continued to intrigue medical scientists and reporters.

In an interview conducted by James D'Eramo *(New York Native,* September 9, 1984), Robert Gallo was asked about my finding of acid-fast bacteria in Kaposi's sarcoma, and about reports from Denmark showing that Dapsone (an anti-leprosy drug) might be successful in the treatment of this form of cancer. Gallo responded, "I don't know the cause of Kaposi's sarcoma. My guess is that is must be related to HTLV-3 infection in some way. Perhaps it's caused by a release of growth factors from HTLV-3 infected cells." D'Eramo than asked why Kaposi's sarcoma occurred mostly in gay men. Gallo remarked, "I don't know. Kaposi's sarcoma confuses me."

Medical scientists continued to downplay the connection between the AIDS virus and the development of Kaposi's sarcoma in gay men with AIDS. With the discovery of the new AIDS virus, even the previous widely-touted connection between the cytomegalovirus and Kaposi's sarcoma was rarely mentioned anymore in scientific papers.

In May 1985, a revealing autopsy study of 52 AIDS cases (23 Haitians, 19 male homosexuals, 5 intravenous drug abusers, 2 hemophiliacs, and 3 persons at unknown risk) *indicated for the first time a very high incidence of Kaposi's sarcoma in AIDS patients of all types.* Early in the epidemic, Kaposi's sarcoma was found in only about one-third of gay men with AIDS. *However, this new autopsy study showed that this form of cancer was present at death in over 94% of AIDS patients!* The report, written by a group of pathologists headed by Lee Moskowitz of the University of Miami School of Medicine, was unique in other aspects. It was the first study to suggest that Kaposi's sarcoma frequently affected the "T-cell" areas of the lymphatic tissue, particularly the lymph nodes and the spleen.

Could this cancerous destruction of immunologically reactive tissue cause immunologic abnormalities in AIDS patients? The pathologists wrote: "The remarkable occurrence of Kaposi's sarcoma in T-cell domains in virtually all of our cases suggests it may play a more important role in the pathogenesis of AIDS than is generally appreciated. We believe that Kaposi's sarcoma contributes to the deterioration of cellular immunity seen in patients with AIDS by invasive destruction of T-cell domains, as in lymphomas or Hodgkin's disease."

Moskowitz's report did not go unnoticed by AIDS watchers. Two important questions were raised. Was the "new" HTLV-3 virus really the *sole* cause of AIDS? *Or was AIDS actually an epidemic of cancer in the form of Kaposi's sarcoma?*

Other 1985 autopsy reports were also illuminating. Kevin Welch, *et al,* studying 36 AIDS deaths in San Francisco, (32 were gay men), discovered that 83% of the deaths were due to opportunistic infection. Twenty five cases had infection with cytomegalovirus. Eight cases suffered from TB infections due to acid-fast mycobacteria. Twenty four cases had a history and/ or post-mortem evidence of Pneumocystis pneumonia.

Another autopsy study of 56 AIDS cases reported by George Niedt and Roger Schinella, pathologists at New York University Medical Center, showed that common bacteria and TB mycobacteria caused serious infections in over half the patients. *These infections were frequently unrecognized and were often undiagnosed by the physicians.* Although these autopsy reports revealed important and disturbing information, the most startling AIDS report of 1985 came out of Belle Glade, in southern Florida.

The big AIDS outbreak in Belle Glade, Florida, suggested that AIDS might not always be a sexually transmitted disease.

Thirty seven AIDS cases reported from this town of 17,000 residents indicated that the small rural community had not only the highest incidence per capita of AIDS in America, but also in the world.

Peculiarly, half the reported cases were *not* homosexual, bisexual, or drug abusers. Some patients did not have a positive blood test for the new HTLV-3 virus. Rather than sexual or drug-related factors, the epidemiologic evidence strongly pointed to socioeconomic factors such as poverty, poor sanitary conditions, and overcrowded living conditions as the cause of the AIDS outbreak. Continuing investigation of these Belle Glade cases will undoubtedly increase our understanding of AIDS as more than a disease simply caused by the new HTLV-3 virus.

Based on many years of microscopic observations, I was certain that AIDS was a form of cancer. At age 78, Dr. Virginia Livingston-Wheeler was continuing to declare that cancer was an infectious disease caused by acid-fast bacteria. Her book, "The Conquest of Cancer" (1984), was creating a furor in the scientific community.

A rather unflattering article on Livingston and her revolutionary ideas about bacteria in cancer appeared in *The Los Angeles Times* (April 6, 1984). For more than twenty years I had been scientifically confirming many of her observations of microbes in cancer and collagen diseases. I entered the brouhaha by allowing myself to be interviewed. I defended her publicly by agreeing with her unorthodox view of the infectiousness of cancer.

Livingston's many scientific opponents were merciless in their condemnation of her life's work in cancer microbiology. Robert Gallo was quoted as saying, "What is going on in this country? This is insanity! She can have her theories and what can I say? I don't know of anything to support it. I can't see any basis and I don't know what to say or what analogy to give you."

Whether or not medical scientists believed Virginia Livingston-Wheeler's idea of a "cancer microbe," she was correct in her belief that cancer was an infectious disease. The death of "the bubble boy" in 1984 proved beyond doubt that cancer could be transmitted between people, at least in the case of David.

There has never been a human being as closely studied by physicians and medical researchers as David, who was born on September 21, 1971. His birth was anticipated by physicians who knew he would be born with a 50-50 chance of having congenital immune deficiency. Babies born with this rare disease rapidly die of fatal infections unless immediately protected within a germ-free environment.

David's mother had already lost a baby boy to this dread disease. This time the doctors were ready to save her newborn child. As planned, David was delivered by cesarean section in order to prevent possibly fatal contact with vaginal bacteria. Seconds after delivery, David was placed in a plastic, germ-free isolator "bubble" where he lived for 12 years.

On October 12, 1983, David was given a bone marrow transplant taken from his 15-year-old healthy sister. Doctors hoped this transplant would improve his immune system and allow him to live a normal life outside the bubble. If all went as planned, the transplanted bone marrow cells would reproduce and grow within David's body, and help to strengthen his immune system.

Four months later, on February 22, 1984, David was dead of cancer. However, this information was not released to the public until more than a year later.

Initial reports of his death were widely circulated in the

medical press. Physicians claimed David died "of heart failure." As late as January 1985, an editorial on the "the Bubble Boy," appearing in the *Journal of the American Medical Association (JAMA),* stated he died "of causes as yet obscure."

David's final autopsy report, released 15 months after his death, revealed he died of a rapidly fatal form of lymphoma-type cancer known as "B-cell immunoblastic sarcoma." How was it possible for a young boy so carefully protected, studied, and monitored daily by expert physicians to die a horrible death of cancer?

Sophisticated immunologic tests of David's tissue at autopsy showed he died from cancer caused by infection due to the Epstein-Barr virus. This virus was traced back to his sister's bone marrow tissue which had been transplanted into David. David's sister was perfectly healthy. She was carrying the virus within her blood stream with no ill effects. But David could not ward off the virus.

According to pathologists, the Epstein-Barr virus caused the cancer which quickly killed David. The evidence was clear-cut. The genetic material found in David's cancerous "B-cells" exactly matched the genetic material found in his sister's Epstein-Barr virus.

To anyone who thought deeply about David's life in the bubble and his death from cancer, it was evident that *cancer could be an infectious disease.* It could be passed from one person to another, at least in transplant material. It could also probably be transmitted in blood which, according to Livingston, always contains infectious cancer bacteria and related, smaller virus-sized elements.

I had always thought Livingston's ideas about cancer were surprisingly simple. Cancer bacteria were always present in the blood and connective tissue of healthy people. They caused no trouble when the immune system was healthy. But these same microbes could cause chronic and fatal diseases, including cancer, in people with weakened or damaged immune systems.

One fact was now certain. There was no such thing as a guaranteed infection-free tissue transplant. With time, physicians would also learn that there was no such thing as blood free from cancer microbes.

With the AIDS epidemic some physicians and patients were concerned about acquiring the AIDS virus from organ transplants, particularly those donated by homosexual men. The question "should homosexuals be organ donors?" was answered by Israel Penn (*JAMA*, November 9, 1984). The case was a young woman who needed a kidney transplant. Her homosexual brother was willing to act as donor. Would it be safe to transplant his kidney? Dr. Penn said no. "Homosexual men could be carrying the AIDS virus and yet be perfectly healthy . . . transplant surgeons make great efforts to avoid transmitting disease from donor to recipient, (therefore) it is wise to exclude homosexual donors."

By 1985 the scientific appraisal of the AIDS epidemic had fostered the general public belief that male homosexuals were carriers of the new plague. Most people thought gays were responsible for spreading AIDS to the rest of the population. Some insurance companies were insisting on testing certain applicants for AIDS antibodies. Life insurance applications from young unmarried men living in big cities with certain ZIP codes were scrutinized carefully and often turned down. In states like California, where mandatory HTLV-3 blood testing was unlawful, the insurance companies were insisting on a "T and B-cell" immunologic test.

The military was determined to rid itself of the AIDS epidemic before it became a major problem in the Armed Forces. The military didn't have to deal with legislators, lawyers, gay rights activists, liberals, and left wingers. The AIDS blood test was available and the military would use it. Testing of the 1.8 million men and women on active duty throughout the world began in October 1985.

AIDS posed a number of serious problems for the military,

even though only 100 military cases of AIDS had been recorded. Personnel to be sent overseas often needed immunizations for various infectious diseases. These immunizations could be dangerous in immunodepressed people, such as potential AIDS virus carriers. Furthermore, seriously wounded men in combat often needed blood. The battlefield was no place to be testing blood for the AIDS virus. For these reasons, soldiers carrying AIDS virus antibodies were not acceptable to the Armed Forces. New recruits testing positive would be rejected from service. Service persons testing positive would be reassigned.

Homosexual servicemen were obviously the most likely group to test positive. The HTLV-3 blood test would no doubt identify these men not only as suspected AIDS carriers, but as gay men as well. Present U.S. military policy explicitly forbids homosexuals from serving in the Armed Forces. According to the military, homosexuality is considered bad for morale, gays are subject to blackmail, and pose grave risks for military security.

Since 1941, over 80,000 service people have been thrown out of the military for homosexuality. Nevertheless, there are an estimated four million gay and lesbian American veterans who have served their country well. Countless tens of thousands have given their lives in times of war.

The military already had a record of cruelty toward servicemen with AIDS. One unfortunate example was 28-year-old Byron Kinne, who had served in the Navy as a medical corpsman for seven years. In June 1985, when it was discovered that he was dying of AIDS, he was discharged without medical benefits by a discharge board who unanimously decided he was homosexual.

According to the *Los Angeles Herald Examiner* (June 27, 1985), Kinne was devastated. "I feel I've given them seven good years of service. What a person does in their bedroom is their own business. I wouldn't be here at a discharge hearing if I didn't get sick. I just want to take some time and live."

But a Navy spokesman reiterated Naval policy: "Homosexuality is incompatible with military life and seriously impairs the accomplishment of the military mission such as mutual confidence, good morale, and active recruitment."

Kinne sued the Navy. In October 1985, Navy Secretary John Lehman finally made an exception and ruled that Kinne could be granted a medical retirement. A week later, Kinne died of AIDS at the Navy Hospital in San Diego.

Harvey Friedman, an attorney specializing in government employment problems, wrote his opinion about Naval policy on AIDS in the *New York Native*, (October 4, 1985). "Naval officials take advantage of military rules providing that sailors found to be homosexual be discharged and stripped of any benefits that they might otherwise be entitled to, despite the fact that they may have served honorably and were suffering from a tragic disease. One U.S. Admiral, through bogus legal means, went so far as to authorize Navy lawyers to threaten a sailor dying of AIDS with incarceration in the brig if he would not divulge the identities of other homosexuals in the Navy known to him."

The inconsistency of military homophobia was exemplified by a story in the *Los Angeles Herald Examiner*, (October 8, 1985), concerning Sgt. Rolf Lindblom, who had been voted Los Angeles Marine of the Year, in 1984. Lindblom, who is gay, told his superior officers he was homosexual and requested an honorable discharge. Strangely, the Marines balked, claiming Lindblom must *prove* he was gay. Lindblom was exasperated. "What they're asking is for me to make official statements that I have practiced homosexuality and committed sodomy. If I were to make these statements they could court-martial me and destroy the character of my discharge."

One could only wonder how the military would handle the many men and women who would test positive for antibodies to the HTLV-3 virus. A hint of what future military AIDS virus testing might be like was evident in a study performed by Robert Redfield, *et al*, published in *JAMA* (October 18, 1985).

A group of forty one HTLV-3 positive patients (34 men and 7 women) with AIDS or AIDS-related complex was studied at the Walter Reed Army Medical Center in Washington, DC. Over one-third (37%) of the group was heterosexual. The doctors concluded that the AIDS virus could be transmitted from male to female, and from female to male. "Receptive anal intercourse was not a requirement for AIDS." In addition, 73% of the group tested positive for cytomegalovirus; 89% were positive for the Epstein-Barr virus.

It was interesting to discover how the military doctors scientifically determined not only the sexual preference of the men in the group, but also the degree of their promiscuity. They were aware that "military patients may be particularly reluctant to admit to certain risk behaviors." Men were classified as gay if there was "any evidence for behavior characteristics suggestive of homosexual activity." All men had anal swabs for gonorrhea as a further test for homosexual activity.

Heterosexual contact was defined as oral-genital, vaginal, or rectal intercourse. Individuals were defined as having "multiple heterosexual contacts if they had more than 50 different heterosexual partners over the past five years."

The researchers also used "trained investigators" to interview "family members and/or acquaintances when available." The scientific paper had the typical military disclaimer. "The views of the authors do not purport to reflect the position of the Army or the Department of Defense." Nevertheless, it was clear the military was perfectly capable of starting a well-organized witch-hunt for homosexuals now that widespread blood testing for AIDS virus antibodies was a reality.

Continuing but limited HTLV-3 testing of female prostitutes in big cities indicated that this group had a high rate of exposure to the AIDS virus. Ten of 25 women in Miami, and five of 92 women in Seattle tested positive. However only about 100 prostitutes had come down with AIDS, according to 1985 CDC statistics. Drug-addicted prostitutes were at the highest risk.

Prison populations were also thought to be at high risk for AIDS. Surprisingly, the number of AIDS cases in male prisoners was not high but was steadily climbing. The first AIDS case found in a California prison was reported in May 1984. A year later, nine more cases were recorded out of a prison population of 48,000.

By June 1983 eighteen inmates in New York prisons and nine in New Jersey prisons had died of AIDS. New York State prisons had the highest number of cases in the country. This was not surprising. New York City was first in the number of AIDS cases, and 85% of all state inmates were from the New York City area. Seventy five percent of the total inmates (32,000) were drug abusers.

By November 1985 over half of the 14,000 Americans officially diagnosed as AIDS had already died. The other half, with few exceptions, would be dead within two years. New York City had 4600 cases; San Francisco, 1600; Los Angeles, 1200; Miami, 500; and Newark, 400. Four states (Idaho, Montana, North and South Dakota) had no reported cases.

Somewhere between one and two million Americans were said to be already exposed to the virus in 1985. Most would remain perfectly healthy. But scientists were predicting that between 5% and 20% of these people would eventually show signs and symptoms of the disease. AIDS experts also claimed that HTLV-3 positive people would be lifelong virus "carriers," having the ability to sexually transmit the disease to others. However, this view was at odds with the fact that the blood test only detected antibodies to the virus. The test did not in any way indicate the virus was "live," or even present.

Some people were devastated by knowing they had a positive antibody test to the AIDS virus. Certain physicians were emphatic in their belief that all high risk persons should be tested. Sex expert Helen Singer Kaplan, Director of the Human Sexuality Program at the New York Hospital, was quoted in the *Star* (October 8, 1985): "Anyone who is at risk should be tested for the AIDS virus, and those who are infected should never have sex again because their bodies are carrying a poison more deadly than cobra venom." She added: "There is no such thing as safe sex. Those who don't stop having sex are a distinct danger to society."

As a physician and also as a human being, I could never bring myself to make such a demand on healthy patients carrying HTLV-3 antibodies. To insist that these people never again experience in any form the warmth and love of sexual contact with another human being would for me simply be too much to ask. Millions of people can't give up cigarettes. Hundreds of thousands are cocaine addicts. How could one ask two million Americans already carrying HTLV-3 antibodies to stop making love?

My AIDS and "pre-AIDS" gay patients were usually too ill to even think about making love. Others who were healthier seemed to find solace in reaching out to other men who were similarly afflicted. These men were honest in their sexual dealings, looking for people who were also "positive," or unafraid. Together they would find expressions of love in a "safe sex" setting.

The world was only beginning to experience the madness of the AIDS epidemic. According to *Time*, (October 28, 1985), Brazil followed the U.S. with 483 reported cases. France had 392 cases, followed by Haiti (377), Canada (323), West Germany (300), and Britain (225). Predictably, Russia and China had no reported cases.

These AIDS statistics were collected by the World Health Organization. Notably absent were cases from ten Central African nations which refused to issue statistics. Medical reports indicated a large number of Africans had already been exposed to the HTLV-3 virus. Twenty percent of the city dwellers in Rwanda were reported to have HTLV-3 antibodies. As in America, most had absolutely no signs or symptoms of AIDS.

Most epidemiologists believed the epidemic started in Africa or in Haiti, and was brought to America by promiscuous, world-travelling gays. Continuing reports from Central Africa left no doubt that African AIDS was predominantly a *heterosexual* disease. The incidence of AIDS in African men and in woman was about equal, and there were few, if any, admitted homosexuals.

Most American scientists were convinced that AIDS was a brand new disease. Yet, I had long suspected that African Kaposi's sarcoma was the same disease as American AIDS with Kaposi's sarcoma. New African reports confirmed my suspicion.

R.G. Downing, *et al,* reporting in the *Lancet* (March 3, 1984), showed that 12 of 16 Zambian patients with Kaposi's sarcoma had abnormal immunologic findings, such as decreased T-cell counts similar to American gay men with AIDS and Kaposi's sarcoma. Positive cytomegalovirus blood tests were found in all patients (16/16). Epstein-Barr virus tests were positive in 15/16; HTLV tests in 13/16. The scientists concluded, *"African patients with Kaposi's sarcoma seem to have an immunologic and virologic profile similar to that seen in American patients with AIDS."*

The high rate of HTLV-3 exposure of Central Africans did not deter African scientists from finding new diseases caused by the AIDS virus. A *new* AIDS-like African disease called "Slim" disease was discovered in Uganda. According to *Lancet* (October 19, 1985), this illness caused extreme weight loss and chronic diarrhea. In fact, "Slim disease" was probably identical to American AIDS-related complex. The reporting doctors stressed the disease was "clearly associated" with heterosexual promiscuity and with the HTLV-3 virus, (even though eight of 71 patients tested negative to the virus antibody). "Promiscuity" was not defined in this study. However, the investigators wrote: "Although the subjects in our study deny overt promiscuous behavior, their sexual behavior is by Western standards, heterosexually promiscuous." I wondered how the African sexual standard would compare to the U.S. Army heterosexual promiscuity standard of more than 50 different sexual partners every five years?

Despite all this evidence, some people were still convinced that the Cuban refugees brought AIDS to America. Others were equally convinced the AIDS virus was deliberately seeded into the gay community, possibly through venereal disease clinics, as a diabolic government plot to rid the country of troublesome and increasingly militant homosexuals.

By 1985 medical scientists no longer considered AIDS a "gay" disease. Nevertheless. CDC statistics continued to show that homosexual or bisexual men were most at risk for AIDS with 74% of the cases recorded.

The safety of the blood supply by the screening out of HTLV-3 contaminated blood virtually eliminated the possibility of contracting AIDS through blood transfusions. Two percent of the AIDS cases had been acquired through transfusion. New purification methods for blood products used by hemophiliacs would now insure the elimination of this risk group which comprised 1% of AIDS cases. As mentioned, Haitians were no longer included as a separate risk group in the CDC's AIDS statistics.

Inexplicably, homosexual intravenous drug addicts continued to be listed in the "homosexual-bisexual" risk group rather than in the drug abuser group. Although it was now clear that all human beings were susceptible to AIDS, the statistics would attest to the inevitable conclusion held by the American public that male homosexual activity was at the root of the AIDS epidemic.

In 1985 a few science writers began to challenge the established view that the HTLV-3 virus was the sole cause of AIDS. Richard Pearce reviewed the work of scientists who claimed that some people with AIDS were already immunodepressed *before* they became infected with the AIDS virus, (Co-factors and AIDS, *New York Native,* May 19, 1985). The researchers thought infectious agents such as *other* viruses, as well as intestinal parasites were necessary "co-factors" in AIDS.

Dr. Joseph Sonnabend, an infectious disease expert who had treated some of the earliest AIDS cases in New York City, was outspoken in an interview published in the *New York Native* (October 7, 1985). "Unlike what Dr. Robert Gallo (of the National Cancer Institute) tells us, we are very far from understanding this disease. Very little is known. The sort of smugness that emanates from the government scientists is offensive, considering what is at stake and what is happening now. The only people who are pleased over this are the ones who've received millions of dollars worth of support, and these are the government scientists and the big medical centers and also the people who really, I think, have missed the boat. These people have an inordinate influence on media accessibility and are responsible, along with many others, for the panic that's going on now — and the disaster. This all comes from ignorance, and ignorance comes from the failure of authorities to inform people."

There were many unanswered scientific questions surrounding the new epidemic, but in the rush to begin testing of large groups of people for the new virus, the problem areas of AIDS research simply went unnoticed by most scientific experts.

For example, rare reports suggested for the first time that there might be a link between AIDS and tuberculosis (TB). According to *Medical World News* (August 26, 1985), New York City public health officials found that TB preceded or followed identification of HTLV-3 infection in more than 100 AIDS cases. Transients and young men were most at risk. According to Dr. Steven Schultz, "As the number of AIDS cases increases in New York City, so does the number of TB cases associated with AIDS."

Another possible link between infectious TB bacteria and the use of "poppers" during sexual activity was suggested by a study of immunodeficient mice, undertaken by P.R. Gangadharam, *et al*, at the National Jewish Center for Immunology and Respiratory Medicine in Denver (*American Medical News*, September 27, 1985). Before AIDS, the inhalation of "poppers" as a sexual stimulant was popular, particularly in the gay community. "Poppers" in the form of an inhalant (isobutyl nitrite) were widely sold in sex shops under the guise of an incense or as a room deodorizer. In the experiment, the immunodeficient mice were exposed to TB bacteria (*Mycobacterium intracellulare*). These acid-fast microbes often produced a TB-like infection which was frequently fatal in AIDS patients. The mice exposed to "popper" fumes were much more likely to develop the TB infections, indicating to the researchers that the inhalation of poppers might be dangerous, especially to those at high risk for AIDS.

A number of media reports were also calling public attention to the view of a few scientists who strongly believed that the "African swine fever virus" might be causing AIDS. These scientists were supposedly encountering opposition and antagonism from government officials who feared that any tie-in between the eating of pork and the AIDS epidemic would be seriously damaging to the pork industry.

I continued to get some of my research work on bacteria in AIDS published in medical journals, although it was increasingly clear to me that medical editors were becoming more and more unresponsive to any research which did not conform to the idea of the new HTLV-3 virus as the sole cause of AIDS. A published paper, co-authored by Dr. Lyon Rowe, showed photographs of bacteria within the skin tumors of Kaposi's sarcoma, along with similar bacteria in lung tissue affected with Pneumocystis pneumonia. We also showed "African eosinophilic bodies" in the Kaposi's sarcoma tumors of two gay and bisexual patients with AIDS, similar to what pathologists had discovered in African cases decades ago.

We expected that someone in the government scientific community might be interested in the AIDS bacteria that we saw so easily in our office microscope. But strangely, there was no comment from any AIDS expert, nor from any other physician.

In my view, the medical community was on the brink of scientific disaster by initiating the widespread testing of individuals for the HTLV-3 virus. Preliminary blood testing already indicated that about 0.5% of the population would be positive. That would ultimately mean that thousands of people would test positive, as well as "false-positive." They would become the new lepers in America. Most would never show signs of the disease AIDS. Nevertheless, their lives would be damaged and in some cases ruined.

I still believed that AIDS was caused by the same microbes that caused cancer. There was now no doubt that a sexually promiscuous lifestyle, or a drug-oriented lifestyle, or both, could bring about an increased risk of cancer and AIDS. How was that so different from a cigarette-smoking lifestyle that causes 126,00 lung cancer deaths yearly in America, as well as serious cardiovascular disease — the number one killer in America?

The scientific world was convinced that the new AIDS virus had brought about the epidemic of AIDS. No one seemed interested in looking for AIDS bacteria which I could see so easily in all the damaged AIDS tissue I had studied. It was also apparent to me that my unorthodox ideas about AIDS and cancer were clearly upsetting to some important people.

Physicians in high office at the medical institution where I had been associated for over 20 years as a dermatologist and cancer researcher, decided this book might be too controversial. In deference to their suggestion, I have expunged all reference to the institution where I am associated.

In my mind there was no doubt that the HTLV-3 virus, (like all viruses), was potentially a very dangerous infectious agent. I had no doubt that it was a sexually transmitted virus, and it was obvious that gay men in big cities had been heavily exposed to it. But I was convinced *the virus was not what was really killing patients with AIDS.*

I was convinced the "cancer microbe" was really the hidden killer in AIDS, just as it was the hidden killer in cancer. In my opinion, the mystery of AIDS was far from solved. Over the past century, the "cancer microbe" has remained the most elusive, mysterious, and enigmatic microbe in the history of medical science. I decided to risk my scientific reputation in an attempt to bring to light the hidden killer in AIDS — the "cancer microbe." I believe the public should know something more about this microbe and its proposed role in devastating diseases, such as AIDS and cancer. This information is vital for our deeper understanding of these two infectious diseases.

For these reasons, "AIDS: The Mystery and The Solution" had to be written.

References

Levy JA, Hollander H, Shimabukuro J, et al: Isolation of AIDS-associated retroviruses from cerebrospinal fluid and brain of patients with neurological symptoms. Lancet 2: 586-588, 1985.

Council on Scientific Affairs: Status report on the acquired immunodeficiency syndrome, human T-cell lymphotropic virus type-III testing. JAMA 254: 1342-1345, 1985.

Poulsen A, Hultberb B, Thomsen K, et al: Dapsone in the treatment of Kaposi's sarcoma. ACTA Derm Venereol 64: 561-563, 1984.

Moskowitz LB, Hensley GT, Gould EW, et al: Frequency and anatomic distribution of lymphadenopathic Kaposi's sarcoma in the acquired immunodeficiency syndrome. Hum Pathol 16: 447-456, 1985.

Niedt GW, Schinella RA: Acquired immunodeficiency syndrome. Clinicopathologic study of 56 autopsies. Arch Pathol Lab Med 109: 727-734, 1985.

Welch K, Finkbeiner W, Alpers, CE, et al: Autopsy findings in the acquired immune deficiency syndrome. JAMA 252: 1152-1159, 1985.

Lawrence RJ: David the "bubble boy" and the boundaries of the human. JAMA 253: 74-76, 1985.

Shearer WT, Ritz J, Finegold MJ, et al: Epstein-Barr virus-associated B-cell proliferation of diverse clonal origins after bone marrow transplantation of a 12-year-old patient with severe combined immunodeficiency. N Engl J Med 312: 1151-1159, 1985.

Redfield RR, Markham PD, Salahuddin SZ, et al: Heterosexually acquired HTLV-III/LAV Disease (AIDS-related complex and AIDS). JAMA 245: 2094-2096, 1985.

Serwadda D, Sewankambo NK, Carswell JW, *et al: Slim disease: A new disease in Uganda and its association with HTLV-III infection. Lancet 2: 850-852, 1985.*

Downing RG, Eglin RP, Bayley AC: *African Kaposi's sarcoma and AIDS. Lancet 1: 478-480, 1984.*

Van de Perre P, Carael M, Robert-Guroff M, *et al: Female prostitutes: A risk group for infection with human T-cell lymphotropic virus type-III. Lancet 2: 524-586, 1985.*

Cantwell AR Jr, Rowe L: *African "eosinophilic bodies" in vivo in two American men with Kaposi's sarcoma and AIDS. J Dermatol Surg Oncol 11: 408-412, 1985.*

MICROPHOTOGRAPHS

The following eight microphotographs illustrate various microscopic appearances of the "AIDS microbe," and the "cancer microbe," as grown in the laboratory, and observed within the diseased tissue of American patients with "classic" and "Gay" Kaposi's sarcoma, and in enlarged lymph nodes from gay men with suspected early "AIDS."

Figures 1-3:   Acid-fast coccoid forms

Figure 4:   An acid-fast bacillus (rod-form)

Figure 5:   "African eosinophilic bodies"

Figure 6:   Acid-fast coccoid forms and Russell bodies

Figure 7:   The evolution of coccoid forms into Russell bodies

Figure 8:   The "cancer microbe" (*Staphylococcus epidermidis*) isolated and grown from a skin tumor of Kaposi's sarcoma

Figure 1

Diagnosis: "Classic" Kaposi's sarcoma (heterosexual man, age 82).
Tissue: Skin tumor of Kaposi's sarcoma

Kaposi's sarcoma in a Jewish man, age 82, who has had skin tumors of the disease for 26 years. This microscopic section of a Kaposi's sarcoma skin tumor of the nose was specially stained for acid-fast bacteria, by use of the Fite stain. The arrows point to purple-stained, tiny, round, coccoid forms within the tumor in the dermis of the skin. The areas marked "V" represent the tiny, newly-formed blood vessels, normally filled with red blood cells during life. The tiny, cancerous blood vessels (V) are each lined with endothelial cells, which are thought to be the cells which become malignant in Kaposi's sarcoma. The inset shows tiny round cocci of *Staphylococcus epidermidis,* a common bacterium cultured from the Kaposi's sarcoma tumor. Note that the size of the cocci cultured from the malignant tumor is similar to the size of the coccoid forms (arrows) observed within the tumor tissue. The tissue cells and bacteria are magnified 1000 times.

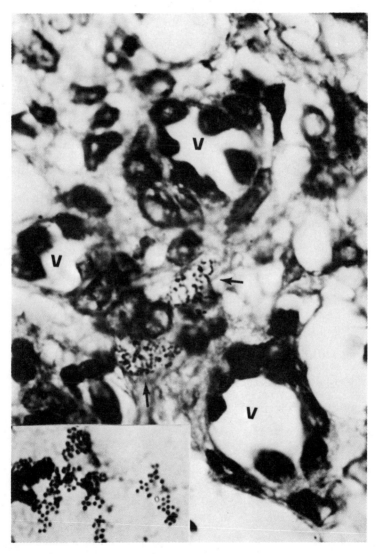

Figure 1

Figure 2

*Diagnosis: AIDS with Kaposi's sarcoma (homosexual man,
        age 29).*
Tissue: Skin tumor of Kaposi's sarcoma

A Fite-stained tissue microscopic section of a skin tumor of Kaposi's sarcoma of the face, of a gay man with AIDS. The tumor appeared on the skin two weeks before the man's death. The arrows point to collections of extracellular coccoid microbial forms within the Kaposi's sarcoma tumor. Note the similarity of these coccoid forms to those found within the enlarged lymph gland of the same patient (Figures 6, and 7). The coccoid forms within the Kaposi's sarcoma tumor of this young gay man are identical to those seen within the "classic" Kaposi's sarcoma tumor of the elderly Jewish, heterosexual man (Figure 1). The tissue is magnified 1000 times.

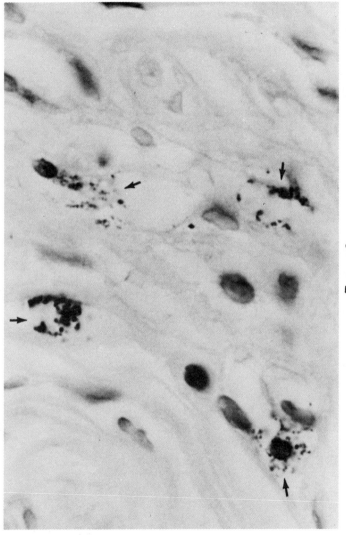

Figure 2

Figure 3

Diagnosis: AIDS with Kaposi's sarcoma (homosexual man, age 32).

Tissue: Skin tumor of Kaposi's sarcoma

A Fite-stained tissue microscopic section of a skin tumor of Kaposi's sarcoma of the leg, of a 32 year-old gay man with AIDS. The arrows point to tiny, intracellular coccoid forms located in the upper dermis portion of the skin. The nucleus (n) of one cell is fairly distinct. Hundreds of densely-packed coccoid forms are surrounding the nucleus. The tissue is magnified 1000 times.

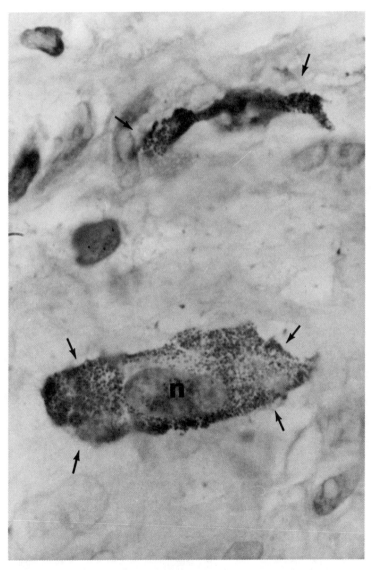

Figure 3

Figure 4

Diagnosis: AIDS with Kaposi's sarcoma (same case as shown in Figure 3).

Tissue: Skin tumor of Kaposi's sarcoma

This Fite-stained section (same section as Figure 3) shows a bacterium appearing as a bright red, acid-fast, rod-shaped bacillus. The bacillus was found in the deep dermis portion of the skin. The finding of acid-fast rods in Kaposi's sarcoma is most unusual, and only two such rods could be detected in examinations of multiple tissue sections of this tumor. This acid-fast rod-form was found in the same tissue section in which thousands of intracellular and extracellular coccoid forms were found (as shown in Figure 3). The tissue is magnified 1000 times.

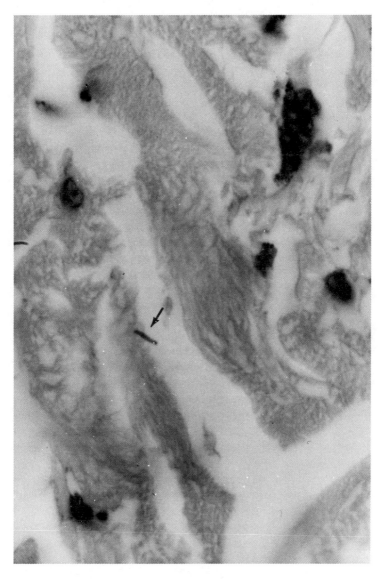

Figure 4

Figure 5

Diagnosis: AIDS with Kaposi's sarcoma (bisexual man, age 51).

Tissue: Skin tumor of Kaposi's sarcoma

This microscopic section was stained with hematoxylin-eosin, the routine stain used by pathologists for tissue diagnosis. The arrows point to pink-stained, tiny, round, "eosinophilic bodies," which were located in and around the tumor cells. These distinct tiny round forms have been observed by pathologists in some African cases of Kaposi's sarcoma. The eosinophilic bodies pictured here are present within the tumor of an American black who has never travelled outside the country. These bodies were also stained with the acid-fast stain indicating that African eosinophilic bodies and acid-fast coccoid forms (as seen in many different forms of cancer, including Kaposi's sarcoma) are one and the same. A vascular slit (VS), normally filled with red blood cells during life, and nearby red blood cells (erythrocytes), labeled "E," are also shown. The tissue is magnified 1000 times.

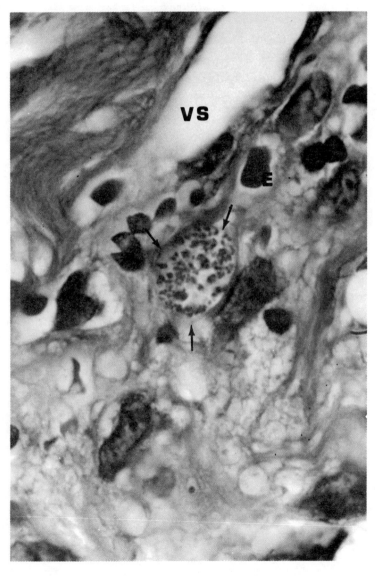

Figure 5

Figure 6

Diagnosis: AIDS with Kaposi's sarcoma (homosexual man, age 29).

Tissue: Lymph node (gland) showing "non-specific hyperplasia"

A microscopic Fite-stained section of an abnormal, enlarged lymph gland, removed one month before the death of a 29 year-old white, gay man with AIDS and Kaposi's sarcoma. The lymph gland was diagnosed as non-specific hyperplasia, by the pathologist. The arrow points to intracellular purple-stained coccoid forms, and nearby large, round, darkly-stained Russell bodies (RB). The size of the tiny intracellular forms (arrow) in the gland is identical to the size of the intracellular and extracellular coccoid forms, discovered in the same man's skin tumor of Kaposi's sarcoma (Figure 2), as well as in the skin tumors of three other men with Kaposi's sarcoma (Figures 1, 3, 4, and 5). The tissue is magnified 1000 times.

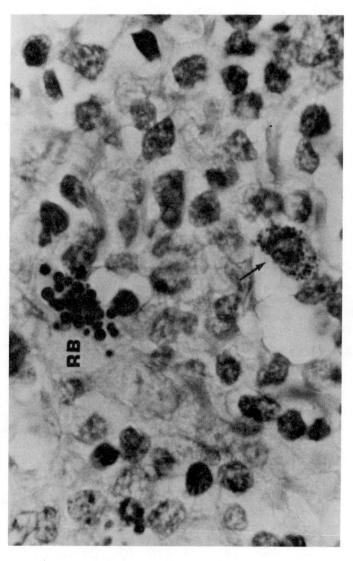

Figure 6

Figure 7

Diagnosis: AIDS with Kaposi's sarcoma (homosexual man, age 29).

   Tissue: Lymph node showing "non-specific hyperplasia"

The same lymph gland as shown in Figure 6. This micropho-tograph shows the transition of tiny, round, extracellular (A) and intracellular coccoid forms (B-D) into progressively larger Russell bodies (E-J) and "giant" Russell bodies (K-L). The forms are magnified 1000 times. (Giemsa stain A-G, J; Fite stain H; Gram stain K, L).

Bacteria in a cell wall deficient state can transform their structure from tiny, round, granular forms into "giant large bodies." It is entirely possible that all the forms shown in this microphotograph are cell wall deficient forms of bacteria.

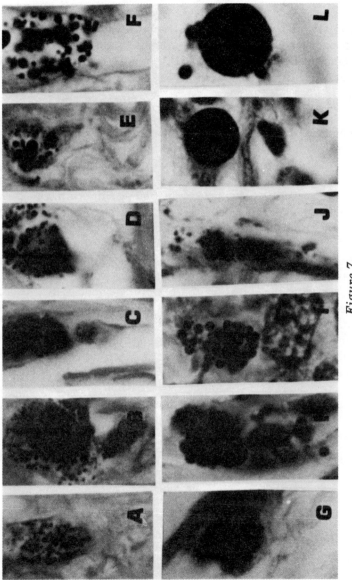

Figure 7

Figure 8

Staphylococcus epidermidis (the "cancer microbe") isolated in bacteriologic culture from a skin tumor of Kaposi's sarcoma (bisexual man with AIDS, age 51 — same patient as described in Figure 5).

This microphotograph shows numerous, tiny cocci of *Staphylococcus epidermidis*, magnified 1000 times. The bacteria were isolated in a liquid medium (thioglycollate broth), and then smeared onto a glass slide for microscopic examination. The microbes on the "smear" were stained with an acid-fast (Ziehl-Neelsen) stain. Two different staining forms of the cocci were identified by this stain. One form (straight arrows) consisted of smaller, purple-stained cocci or "granules." The other form consisted of slightly larger cocci (curved arrows) staining light-pink, indicating that these cocci are weakly acid-fast. The staphylococci are similar in size to the coccoid forms seen in tumors of Kaposi's sarcoma (Figures 1-3). The larger pink-stained staphylococci are also similar in size to the "eosinophilic bodies," which were observed within the same patient's skin tumor (Figure 5). These larger cocci are also comparable in size to certain of the small-size "Russell bodies," as shown in Figures 6 and 7. All human beings normally harbor *Staphylococcus epidermidis*, and this microbe is normally present on the surface of the skin. As mentioned in the text, one form of the cancer microbe is identical to commonplace staphylococci widely distributed in nature. (Bacteriologic culture courtesy of J. E. Jones).

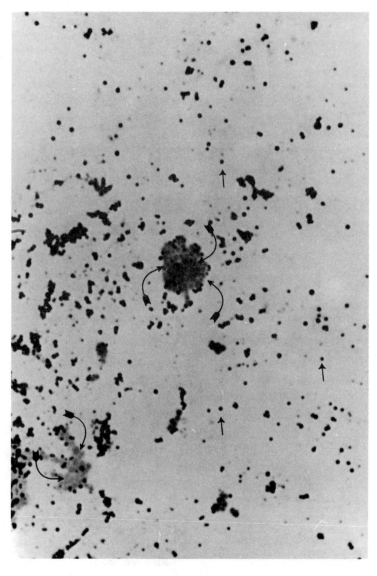

Figure 8

SUBJECT INDEX

INDEX OF PROPER NAMES